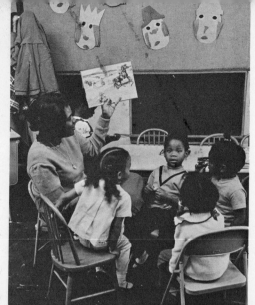

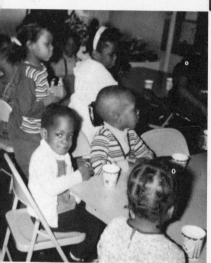

9226 KERCHEVAL: The Storefront That Did Not Burn

9226

Kercheval

The Storefront That Did Not Burn

Nancy Milio

Ann Arbor   The University of Michigan Press

Book design by Quentin Fiore

To the people at Mom and Tots:

Willy Conley
Pat Edwards
Georgianne Evans
Mary Grigsby
Tim Heard
Janice Hicks
William Hitt
Clara Howze
Gwendolyn Hudson
Victoria Jackson
Rosa Lee King
Frank Lewis
Brenda McConnell
Tommie Miller
Martha Prescod
Dorothy Smoot
Rudene Walker
Carolease Wallace
Ann Washington
Judy Weliver
Margie Williams
Gilbert Williams

Acknowledgments

Recreative as it was for me to write this book, it was also an awesome undertaking. And so, in addition to those to whom this work is dedicated, I must also thank certain special people for their constant aid and comfort, Joan Mulligan and Judy Odiorne; for their inspiring ways and thought-evoking criticism, Jim Guinan, Hugh Whipple, and Peter Lallos; for his patient reading and important suggestions, William Himelhoch; for their views as administrators, Margaret Arnstein and Sylvia Peabody; and for many other essentials, my parents.

Nancy Milio
Summer 1969

Contents

Focus

This is the story of a venture in the ghetto, of the development of a ghetto health project which still lives, and of its meaning as I saw it as director. It is a tale told twice, in alternating sections: first as a factual account of events, then as a personal interpretation of those events—the story from the inside of the white outsider who was present. The factual account is indicated in the book by a ruled margin.

The unfolding is literally and allegorically a story of involvement and change, the evolution of a new institution and of the people who made it. It is, in its parallel construction here, the public and private stories behind a benignly named storefront in a Detroit ghetto, the Mom and Tots Center, and of the inevitable intertwining of the two.

It speaks to those who are seeking a way to make a dent in the world, a dent to jar it into something more healthful and whole. It is not intended as a "how-to-do-it" text. That it cannot be. It is a story of what happened in a particular place at a particular time in the contemporary history of the city.

This book does say at least two things. First that health, as quality of life, as "wholeness, unfolding," must be mirrored in the *process* of undertakings intended to improve health. And that those who would involve others, especially the poor, in the process of healthful change, must themselves be involved: the one who would change others must himself be changed.

Prologue

Health is wholeness, unfolding:

It is sharing, significantly, increasingly,
       in the varieties of human experience:
    physically, in the range of activities
      in which the human body can engage;
      not only aggression, but also conciliation,
      not only the proprieties, but also the singularities,
      not only to exhaustion, but also to the crest of vitality;
    sensually, in the possibilities of sensation;
      not confined to extremes:
          rage and excitement, passivity, suppression;
          nor to pain:
          the pain of separation,
          the fear of aloneness;
      but knowing the quiet depths, the tenderness, the nu-
          ances flowing from tones, textures, odors, flavors;
          the joy of well-being, of union and reunion,
          the awesomeness of intimacy;
    culturally, socially, in the designs for living,
      across time and across the world:
      ways of talking, eating, dressing, pleasuring;
      ideas of beauty, of truth, of rightness.
It is growing in awareness:
    of sharing, significantly;
    of self;
    rising above existence, beyond time and space,
      the uniqueness of man.
And it is feeling good about it all, coming into Self-hood:
    expressing one's inner power,
    articulating one's reason-for-being,
    accepting one's sexuality,
      and interdependence:
      receiving and giving,

holding on and letting go,
following and guiding.
Toward wholeness:
responding to the possibilities and limitations of human
experience,
reciprocating, resting, resurgent again;
exploring, discovering,
opening, unfolding,
from diffuseness toward coherence,
simplicity toward complexity,
disparity toward complementarity,
vagueness toward decisiveness,
confusion toward understanding,
toward wholeness.

1
Search for Coherence

. . . The Negro baby born in America today, regardless of the section of the nation in which he is born, has about one-half as much chance of completing high school as a white baby born in the same place on the same day, one-third as much chance of completing college, one-third as much chance of becoming a professional man, twice as much chance of becoming unemployed, about one-seventh as much chance of earning $10,000 a year, a life expectancy which is seven years shorter, and the prospects of earning only half as much.

. . . Difficulties over segregation and discrimination exist in every city, in every state of the Union, producing in many cities a rising tide of discontent that threatens the public safety. . . .

We are confronted primarily with a moral issue. . . .

. . . A great change is at hand, and our task, our obligation, is to make that revolution, that change, peaceful and constructive for all. . . .

JOHN F. KENNEDY
June 11, 1963
Television Address to the People

The intersection of Kercheval and McClellan Streets in Detroit
is America at the crossroads:

Corner drugstore, a stern light-skinned Negress the pro-
    prietor, a "White Nigger" they called her,
Bank,
Cleaners,
Allan Temple, brick faced, once Baptist,
    now Christian Methodist Episcopal,
Barber shop,
Grocery,
Day-old bakery,
Dime store,
Laundromat,
Tree of Life Church, a storefront,
    and next door,
ACME, Adult Community Movement for Equality,
    active behind its boarded-up headquarters.

Interspersed, are
Vacant storefronts—
    the owners live somewhere on the white fringe
    of the city—
Broken bottles, especially on Monday mornings,
Beer cans,
And a variety of trash spilling over
    from the alley running parallel to McClellan.

Surrounding it, are
Tightly packed two- and four-family flats,
Most more than fifty years old,
Now officially judged among the least desirable in
    the city.[1]

The people who live there are Blacks, once called Negroes,
    Colored, and Niggers.
And they are poor:
In money,
Space,
Schooling,

Health,
And the chances to do much better.[2]

They have more children than other Detroit families
And there are more old people;
But their babies are dying faster,
And more of their old people are dying of chronic
    diseases.[3]

But on a warm day Kercheval is alive:
Teenagers are thumping in time to soul music;
The young boys tease and fight;
The young men, out of work for whatever reason,
    saunter in two's and three's in the sun;
Old men, the hope of work long gone,
    sit on corner stoops,
    drinking beer.

Women,
    carrying groceries or laundry or children,
    enjoy the air,
    wave to a neighbor,
    stop to glance in the Thrift Shop window.

A sudden chill covers the street:
    faces fall blank and cold,
    motion is subdued
Whenever The Big Four,
    in their black squad car
    ride slowly along.

Kercheval was dark and quiet. Snow was falling. It was the last night of January, 1966. Most people were keeping warm indoors. About a dozen women and a couple of young men from ACME, the Adult Community Movement for Equality, were gathering in one of their houses. That meeting was more than three years in the making.

*   *   *   *   *

For years, various groups had been meeting to express their concern over what was happening on the lower Southeast Side. As early as 1960, the Eastern Community Council, ECC, formed

> to provide a way for all Block Clubs in the Council area to get to know one another, share ideas, and work together to make the Council community the best possible place to live and work. . . .
>
> to provide a forum for clubs to talk over problems. . . .
>
> to promote better understanding and cooperation between the community and our schools. . . .
>
> to have a continuing concern for youth, urban renewal, neighborhood conservation, improved housing, police-community relations. . . . health and sanitation problems. . . .

(And)

> On controversial questions, the Council shall take no action in its own name, but present both sides of the issue in a fair and impartial manner. . . . The Council shall be nonsectarian, nonpartisan, and nonpolitical. . . .[4]

Then came the Great Cities School Improvement Project

> to develop academic and social competence in each child in spite of his limited background.[5]

And then the Presbyterians and Episcopalians began

> a sector strategy, . . . organizing their churches in the eastern sector of the city to explore the possibilities of suburban-inner city involvement in the problems of the poor.[6]

And after them, the Citizens Committee of Consolidated Block Clubs formed.

And after them, the East Side Improvement Association (ESIA) organized to

> improve the physical and moral environment, . . . eliminate nuisances or unwholesome influences, cooperate with various city departments in improving the health, safety, physical, economic, and cultural standards of residents. . . . develop neighborliness in seeking common objectives.[7]

They had no reluctance about exerting pressure on City Hall, and they did, but using only "proper" channels.

And then people from all those groups waged a campaign in 1963 to have their community, among five others, designated a Neighborhood Conservation Area by the City. The aims were

> to conserve the structures and other physical elements and to stabilize the population for the insurance of an orderly and desirable social environment.[8]

But the community was bypassed in favor of an area farther from the center of the city.

In their homes families lived with the problems community groups were trying to solve.

There was Vera Watkins:
About forty,
Pleasantly shapeless,
Nine years of schooling in Alabama,
before and during the cotton fields,
Mother of seven:
Carolyn, sixteen years,
Teddy, fourteen,
Gregory, ten,
Arletha, eight,
Marvin, seven,
Marcella, four,
And Deneen, two months,
born prematurely, about three and a half pounds.

Her husband, James,
Almost sixty,
Worked as a cook from 6 A.M. to 2 P.M.,
And then as a run-way hand at the airport
from 3 P.M. to midnight.

Not quite enough money to pay the obstetrician
at the nearest clinic,

And often not enough time to go downtown
to the City clinic.
If enough time,
      then no one to stay with Marcella,
      or no ready transportation;
The same for getting to the Immunization Clinic.
The same for getting the birth-control pills
she wanted.
And on the day she planned to go,
      Gregory might have an asthma attack,
      or get another cut under his eye,
      or on his hand.

Not quite enough money
      for a new car,
      or new TV,
      or new curtains,
      or new clothes,
      or steak.
But enough
      for secondhands;
      for chicken wings,
      and neck bones,
      liver and onions,
      and pinto beans,
      green beans,
      and homemade cornbread;
And love and noise,
      laughter and tears,
And church
And hospitality.

They lived with
      the homemade and tentative repairs
         on the toilet
         and on the cupboard door;
Mr. Watkins never did get the back steps fixed,
      or put a lock on that back door—
         until they'd had two robberies.

There was Johnnie West:
Big,
Black,
And beautiful, literally;
A few years out of a Tennessee high school,
A few months out of a downtown night spot,
A new mother of baby Grace,
*   six pounds, four ounces.*

Her husband was tall,
Handsome,
Jealous,
And used a controlling hand on her.
He was a shoe clerk.

Their apartment: three rooms, small;
No phone,
Little light,
Leaking faucets,
Used furnishings,
Many books.
And filled with dreams:
Of a house,
A job to satisfy her,
College for Grace,
Travel,
Someday.

Looking to the future:
She managed to get the coil put in
*   for birth control;*
But who could she trust to keep Grace
*   while she looked for a job—*
*   so she could keep a job?*

And there was Mertus Butler.
Short, small, talkative;
A year of college before men and money problems
*   helped her flunk out;*

A glass eye (it helped her fail a civil service physical)
    and a few scars;
Two babies, the latest premature, Anisa;
    two fathers,
Several jobs,
Many more applications,
Now Welfare.
Her upper flat, in the rear
Was in perpetual upheaval
With an array of visitors,
Sitters,
House bugs,
Dogs,
Preschooler Kay,
Piles of clothes,
And playthings,
And debris.
She pursued ideas
As readily and wildly
As men.

And then the War on Poverty moved into Detroit. It was known as the Mayor's Committee for Total Action against Poverty (TAP). Its Community Action Programs were to combat poverty by

> developing employment opportunities, improving human performance, motivation and productivity, or bettering the conditions under which people live, learn, and work; . . . conducted with maximum feasible participation of members of the areas and groups served. . . .[9]

Its first battles were fought on the West Side, beginning in 1965.

At that time, the *Detroit News* reported:

> In the plans of the more militant civil rights groups in Detroit, the issues of housing, education, and jobs will take a back seat

this summer. Instead, they'll concentrate on politics. Their aim is to create new pressure groups by organizing Detroit's slum dwellers into political units. . . .

The change is a response to the stirrings caused by the black nationalist movement represented in Detroit by the Freedom Now Party and the Black Muslims. . . .

(One such group is) A C M E. . . . A field project of the Detroit Branch of the Northern Student Movement (N S M). (The white N S M head said that A C M E) is not seeking to strike a compromise with city officials but rather seeking a . . . "transformation of this entire society." N S M is a force for continuing agitation. . . .

(The Mayor's office stated) "Much of the steam can be taken out of protest attacks by granting some of the demands. It's the 'kill it with kindness' approach. . . .

"We've got a funny town. Most of the Negro community is a bystander to all this militant stuff. The really extreme groups don't seem to be taking anyone with them. All the big issues like housing and schools are going largely untouched by the legitimate civil rights organizations."[10]

A C M E, the Adult Community Movement for Equality, with the support of N S M leaders, the Northern Student Movement, submitted its proposal to T A P for an antipoverty program on the lower Southeast Side:

The Poverty bill talks about poor people participating in decision-making and so does T A P. But decisions for T A P are made by a committee which includes only one Negro and which does not include any poor people. . . . We do not believe that T A P is serious about eliminating poverty. We in A C M E are serious—we make the following proposals:
First we require an end to discrimination which keeps Negro wages only one-half that of whites, and leaves twice as many Negroes unemployed as whites.

I. Administration:

    A. The Community will run the poverty program. Poor people will be paid to decide:

      1. how to end poverty,

      2. what jobs need doing,

      3. who will do them.

   B. One representative from each block will serve on the body.

II. Jobs:

   A. Training programs will be tailored to community needs as determined by the representatives, i.e., home remodeling.

   B. Everyone trained will be guaranteed a job or an adequate income.

III. Housing:

Everyone will get low-cost housing which fits their needs.

IV. Education:

   A. Free textbooks and newspaper and magazine subscriptions for each family who wants them.

   B. First-rate schools and teachers for all.

   C. Reduce classes to fifteen members.

   D. Begin preschool program in a neighborhood building or house.

   E. Establish neighborhood reading centers.

   F. Hire teaching assistants from the community.

V. Recreation:

   A. Adequate recreation facilities close to home for all ages.

   B. Trained supervisors hired from the community.

VI. Medical Care:

All necessary medical care will be provided free to those in need.

VII. Legal Assistance:

   A. Educate people to their rights and responsibilities.

        B. Provide free lawyers.

VIII. Voting:

        A. Register people in their homes.

        B. Educate people to their political power.[11]

ACME, feared by other community groups, nevertheless went with the East Side Improvement Association, the Eastern Community Council, and others to meetings with TAP field staff. In three months three successive elections of officers took place in an effort to form a cohesive group. By April, 1965, ACME walked out, angrily.

Meanwhile, a young community health nurse had drawn up a modest proposal for the Visiting Nurse Association (VNA) which embraced some of the concerns of these neighborhood groups and the personal problems of her patients—people like Vera Watkins, Johnnie West, and Mertus Butler. Her goal, as stated in the project proposal, was

> to reduce the deterrents to maternal and child care, namely, those of transportation and accessibility of services, supervision and dependent children, and insufficient motivation and lack of knowledge.

> A decentralized facility, such as a storefront, or suitable house (which would serve as a neighborhood center) would reduce the transportation problem by providing a prenatal clinic in association with a central-city hospital, . . . a family planning service, . . . well-baby care, including immunizations, . . . a cooperative transportation service, . . . a cooperative babysitting service or day-care center (part-time), . . . and group teaching. . . .

> In recognition of the socio-economic problems which, as perceived by families, often take priority over health needs, the proposed Center would provide space for neighborhood groups to cope with local problems as they define them. . . .

> The specific forms should be left to the needs and wishes of the neighborhood. . . .

Ideally, an additional person (preferably a Negro) oriented to grass-roots community organization would be specifically hired to promote and coordinate the nonpublic health aspects of the Project and to explore new ways of mobilizing the resources of people in a neighborhood setting. . . .[12]

Early in 1965 the VNA had submitted this proposal to the Mayor's poverty program, as the only possible source for funds and official support.

A white supporter of the Northern Student Movement, knowing of ACME's interests and frustrations, arranged an unofficial meeting between the author of the proposal and Wilson Brown, the leader of ACME. The purpose was to get ACME's opinion of the project. Wilson, a slim Black with a small mustache, called his female cochairman, Jancie; they agreed to read the proposal.

Then came the Selma Incident in Alabama—where police dogs were unleashed on peaceful civil rights demonstrators—and a Protest March in downtown Detroit, and a two-day train to Washington to urge passage of the pending Civil Rights Bill. ACME and NSM, as well as others from the lower Southeast Side, were there.

Two weeks later the Proposal hadn't been read. Wilson and some others complained about their frustrating discussions with TAP. Give them another week.

In the meanwhile TAP had approved the VNA Project and would provide funds on July 1.

Back at ACME, a week later, the Proposal was still not read. Jancie's husband had forced her to resign her chairmanship because she had gone on the Washington train. Wilson said to contact Jeannie, another ACME woman.

Two weeks later Jeannie was barbecuing ribs in the alley behind ACME. "Oh ya, Wilson said you got something going. . . ." With that, she called another woman, Tonya, and they agreed to set up a meeting to discuss the project in two weeks, May 26.

Two other women in the neighborhood had been making plans for the day-care program. One, Mrs. Queen, was a former teacher, and wife of a teacher, a Negro, soft-spoken, refined, quietly interested. The other, Elma Hill, was a Scotland-born wife of a minister, a former social worker; quick, intelligent, well educated. The plan was that they would share the responsibility for supervising the program.

On May 25 TAP telephoned that no budgetary funds were available for the Neighborhood Center Project (officially designated Maternity Satellite Center). A new proposal was required to go to the Office of Economic Opportunity in Washington, the central agency in the poverty fight.

The next day, in a thunder shower, the ACME women met at Tonya's house. There were five. They heard the news about the loss of money. "Wouldn't you know it! The mother fuckers!"

They talked about the Center, especially the day-care program. Couldn't the program be ten hours, full-time, so mothers could work? Then they could pay a fee. Mothers who didn't work could volunteer their time.

Could there be some way to teach the teen-age girls about sex?
Could the girls be hired as babysitters?
When would it start?
No one knew, now.

In the months of waiting that followed, the cry for Black Power began to be heard more often across the country. Into Detroit came the national director of the Northern Student Movement, now a Black. He delivered a speech to the local membership:

> The civil rights movement has ignored that 'other' America. It has functioned as though the Negro was and wished only to be a dark-skinned white man. And even if some secretly hold to that belief, the country does not. To the country one is merely a nigger. A nigger has no sex, no humanity, no brothers or sisters or family. It bleeds but knows no pain, it hungers but need not eat. It does not matter. This is the truth of black existence in America which the movement avoids. . . .

> Any institution in the country—police, schools, etc.—any institution in the society is founded on two central premises:

White supremacy and staying in power. White people have more power than black because the society recognizes them. Democracy more or less works for white people, but it does not work for black. The American institutions irrespective of the stated purpose seek to protect themselves. . . .

What NSM is doing now is beginning to raise what seems to us to be the true question of attempting to build a movement on *our* experience, on the black reality, a movement which is *ours*. . . . When that movement is formulated and cohesive, then those white people who are serious can be allies. . . . We're not concerned about people who want to support the black struggle out of friendship. . . . You come to work in the struggle, (then) . . . you come to work on the terms of the organization.

Black people have to give up that myth of the good white man, for as long as they cling to the myth of the good white man, they have an excuse for not struggling themselves. . . .[13]

And so white people left NSM. They formed the Friends of NSM to

communicate with the ghetto-based movement, to support and interpret its efforts, and take initiative action in our own communities in confronting others on the issue of racism. . . .[14]

After January, 1966, white supporters were no longer seen at ACME, although their funds continued to sustain it. A new chairman arrived from the East to take Wilson's place. He was Luke Pride.

Word came from OEO at the end of 1965 that the Maternity Satellite Center would receive funds by February, 1966. Once again, the Friends of NSM helped set up a meeting with ACME's chairman at ACME headquarters.

The ACME store front served as communications center, meeting place, training ground, and limited living quarters. It had two desks, a gas burner, a dozen folding chairs, some makeshift bookshelves, and stacks of mimeographed speeches and pamphlets. Its plasterboard walls were covered with city maps, pictures and words of Malcolm X, and news clippings of police incidents.

Luke Pride was soft-spoken but incisive. He said ACME was no longer merely going to protest police brutality. It was going to work to develop a strong identity in black people, especially the young people. This was why ACME was interested in preschool.

This was why he liked the idea of a day-care program in the Maternity Satellite Center. But why not hire a man for the day-care program? And why not a Negro health worker to head the Center, instead of a white community health nurse?

He was told if he could find such people, they would be hired. But he knew that just then such people were not visible.

He would think about involving ACME women in the Center. He would think about men who could renovate a building for the Center. Give him a week.

A week later, the storefront was closed. No one answered the phone for three days.

Jeannie on her own agreed to a meeting in her apartment. No one was there on the appointed evening.

The next morning she answered the phone. Yes, her grandmother had died and she just didn't feel like talking, so she didn't answer the buzzer.

Other women, like Vera Watkins, Johnnie West, and Mertus Butler thought the neighborhood needed something for children; a place to keep them off the street, a place to prepare them for school. They would be willing to work on it. Mertus had a myriad of questions and started talking to friends. Mrs. Watkins reacted this way, "Now wouldn't that be somethin'. . . . But I never worked before. . . . Who'd hire me to take care of kids anyway?"

The ACME office was open again. Luke hadn't thought of anyone to do the renovations. But he did know a man who could use the money, Pete Collins. He had no phone, but Luke knew *about* where he lived, three blocks away. No, he couldn't make the contact himself because they weren't on speaking terms. Of course ACME meant what it said about wanting to have a voice in planning programs for the community! He called Jeannie and arranged a meeting that evening.

Two little girls in the vicinity of Pete Collins' house had never heard of anyone by that name. They eventually went into a corner flat with broken steps. Their mother came to the door. She listened when she heard that Luke Pride thought Pete Collins might want a contracting job. She agreed to have her husband call—although it would have to be after 11 P.M., since he was working. And, his business name was Pete Collins Jackson.

Pete Collins Jackson called. He was interested.

Jeannie thought the Center was worth talking over with more A C M E women next week, on January 31.

Mertus Butler, Johnnie West, and Mrs. Watkins would attend the meeting, too.

Mrs. Queen would not be able to go; she thought it best for her family if she went back to college for a teaching certificate, *officially* to qualify her as a teacher.

Elma Hill knew, sadly, that for most people who would meet on the thirty-first, the fewer with white skin, the better. So she would not be going.

*   *   *   *   *

On that last night of January, 1966, they arrived, one or two at a time, in the snow, at Jeannie's mother's house. Mertus brought two friends, Mrs. Robinson and Mrs. Jefferson; they came in the new Jefferson station wagon, since Mertus' old coupe couldn't be counted on to get through the snow. Jancie, Tonya, and a few other ACME women came too. Johnnie never came; she had lost the address. In all, there were twelve.

Luke listened from the dining room. He thought ACME women could help, but he wasn't sure whether they should be hired by the Center.

The ACME women, most of them in slacks, sat in one-half of the living room.

The preliminary conversation was lively, although some had never met before. It ranged from the rise and fall of block clubs (Mrs. Watkins said nothing; she remembered how ACME people had frightened the club on her block out of existence), to stories about "getting caught" and how they wished birth-control pills were available *then*, to poking fun at the Freedom Movement:

> I dreamed one night that the Lord called me to go to Selma.
> And I said, "But Lord I'm afraid."
> "It's your responsibility," said the Lord.
> "Lord, I'm afraid."
> "Then I'll go with you."
> "Then I'll go, Lord—but only as far as Cincinnati!"

So Mrs. Jefferson decided not to go to Selma.

Some of their jokes were not for an outsider to understand. It seemed best not to laugh at experiences which only those who had lived them could rightfully satirize.

The meeting turned to the day-care program. Everyone agreed that it would help their children "grow up to be what we want them to be," an aim having many meanings among them. They wanted an all-day program, but not enough Poverty Program funds were budgeted for that.

> Well if we can't have an all-day program now, it should start later in the morning so's mothers can get the other children off to school.

> The clinic should be after lunch and be over before the children come home from school.

> Why don't we have clubs for the older children after school?

> Mack is a good street for it, or Kercheval, wherever it's easy for mothers to get to. (The empty storefront on Kercheval across from A C M E seemed as good as any.)

> We all could make curtains to decorate the place.

> What's it going to be called? I wouldn't know what 'Maternity Satellite Center' means. It has to say what's in it, so's mothers will know. . . . What about 'Mom and Tots'? The Mom and Tots Center.

The stuff which makes for life had congealed, at least for the moment.

To me, Kercheval

and McClellan streets represent more than the ongoing tragedy of the American city. They intersect an area where many South European families once lived, and where I lived as a little girl. This was the neighborhood my parents, second-generation Italians, moved away from so that their two children could grow up in a newer, and, in their eyes, better community.

I saw the neighborhood again after college, as a nurse in the Visiting Nurse Association. It had "changed." In the homes of the Negro families whom I visited I saw a world that I had not known existed. I *felt* that other world. And I knew I was not getting through to the people.

This awareness that we were talking past each other instead of to each other distressed me. Under these circumstances, how could I be effective? How could I teach them anything about health? At the time I thought I knew enough about the meaning of health to teach it. Wasn't that what I was educated for?

The communication problem had not been there when I visited white families on the suburban fringe. My intentions were the same here. What was wrong? I wondered whether other community health nurses had met the same problem. What had they done about it? I was told not to get upset, to just do the best I could; you couldn't change "these people."

After fourteen months I went elsewhere in another kind of community health work. There I visited families of all income levels throughout the metropolitan area. There I worked with professional workers and laymen at many organizational levels in a variety of health and welfare agencies. I experienced the city in a broader framework. I could see how people in one part of the city were living in inhuman circumstances in contrast to those in another part of the city. I wanted to help eliminate the disparity.

I believed in this possibility. Even though I'd had difficulty communicating with poor black people, I had done so, if only rarely. I had seen in their eyes moments of profound pain and sorrow, softness and joy. There had been moments of wordless understanding between us. I knew it was possible. I wanted to find a way to make it *readily* possible, between individuals and between the black and white, the affluent and the indigent of the city.

I began my search with a traditional orientation, seeking answers in school and church. In a graduate school evening course I first heard about "community organization," people as a group finding answers to problems as they themselves define the problems. This seemed to me a natural approach for community health. I scoured the literature, but found nothing on community organization and public health. I wrote a paper to clarify my own thinking. In it I sketched an outline of how health and welfare professionals in Detroit could work with groups of people in their neighborhoods, beginning with the problems the people are concerned about. It seemed impossible that I could ever have a chance to try such a thing in a period when poverty and the urban crisis had not yet captured widespread attention.

At the same time, I got involved in a variety of community organization efforts, first on the West Side of the city, and then, when I had the opportunity, on the East Side, in the Kercheval-McClellan neighborhood. Most of these efforts, whether through churches or schools, city government or independent block clubs, failed to have much lasting impact on the people involved or on their surroundings. Many were superficial, controlled by professionals, and short-lived. Even the people who joined block clubs, although with relatively low incomes, were not typical of the neighborhood. Only 11 percent of them received welfare grants, their average education was more than nine years, and they were homeowners who had lived in Detroit more than ten years. And, they engaged in very little political activity.[15]

But through these efforts which budded, struggled, and died, lines of communication formed among neighborhood-oriented professional people in the schools, churches, and social agencies and concerned residents of the neighborhood, even though these residents were not usually those for whom all these well-intentioned groups were being formed.

And with each failure, the tenor of emerging groups changed. They became more militant and radical in both their goals and the means they advocated to reach their goals. There was a stark change from the school-church-city supported organizations of 1960 to ACME in 1966. Yet even ACME, as militant as it was thought to be, attempted to introduce its ideas by the means prescribed by TAP; nevertheless, they were unable to do so because of the fears and misgivings of older and more traditional neighborhood groups, many of whose leaders considered themselves political liberals. Then, too, the strategy of the Mayor's office to grant minor requests rather than deal with basic issues contributed to an emerging militancy.

These activities became for me, in effect, a training ground in community organization. But I still sought a way to be involved in neighborhood organization in my day-to-day work, for individual nurse-patient activities could not deal with the fundamental problems of the ghetto. Graduate work in neither social work, nursing, nor public health offered what I wanted. Besides, I did not want to return to school for two years even to become officially "qualified."

Finally, someone in the Visiting Nurse Association read the paper I had written on community organization and public health, and I was asked, "Why don't you come back here and do what you want?" So in May, 1963, I did, with the understanding that my district as a visiting nurse would include the Kercheval-McClellan neighborhood.

I was assigned to work in the affluent suburbs of the far East Side—because the nurse then working in the Kercheval district did not want to relinquish that area. For six months I worked in the suburbs and as before spent my evenings and weekends with the neighborhood groups around Kercheval.

My naiveté at the time about the politics of living, the use of power, the force of vested interests, was immense. I believed in the efficacy of the helping professions, medicine, nursing, teaching, social work. I accepted their credos at face value, and I believed in their organizations and agencies. I thought that the aims of well-intentioned professionals were as a matter of course carried out through established institutions. Consequently, I thought I was being fairly astute when I determined that if there was any place in Detroit where a community health nurse would get a chance to do what I wanted to try, it would be the VNA, which has the reputation of being a very stable, respectable, solvent, and charitable home health care agency, the second largest of its kind in the country. Two and a half years out of college, and I was not able to think of myself outside the category of "nurse." I was not a person with an idea and a will and a heart; I was a professional person with an idea, working within the understandable limitations of an organizational setting.

What I had heard as a promise from the VNA to "do what you want to do" was forgotten by the VNA.

In the fall of 1963 I was reassigned to the Kercheval-McClellan area to do the regular visiting nurse service of caring for the sick in their homes, and calling on new mothers and babies. My involvement with neighborhood groups continued in the evenings and on weekends.

I was still optimistic as I began working officially in the Kercheval area. I was going to be the best community health nurse I could be, using the individual patient-visit approach, until I could find some way of working directly with community groups. That could not be done "on agency time" because I had "nothing concrete." My supervisor agreed to help when I asked her to alter the district boundaries to coincide with block club areas; but four months later, I myself had to do the clerical work to implement that change.

My personal diary reflects my feelings just prior to going back to Kercheval-McClellan. I wrote, "Tonight I saw the New York Philharmonic and Leonard Bernstein: his work seems as exhilarating to him as each person's chosen way of life ought to be." But after working in the neighborhood's homes three weeks —although the days were "fascinating"—they were also "exhausting and frustrating. . . . I am uncertain about my direction. . . . How shall I work out my ideas? And do I have anything worth working out?" In the months that followed I tried all the traditional methods that health professionals are supposed to use to improve people's lives—working with clinics, visiting teachers, social workers, welfare workers; holding interagency conferences to discuss "multiproblem families." I wrote, "The days are almost overwhelming as I see more and more how almost impossible some circumstances are for resolution. . . . Working with individual families only emphasizes how inadequate present means are, only reinforces my certainty for the path I'm taking. . . . Sometimes the direction gets so foggy, and there's no guarantee that someday the frustrations will end. . . ."

Working in the neighborhood, I tried to proselytize within the V N A as well, leading inservice education conferences, writing articles, raising questions: Why are we doing what we're doing? What are we accomplishing? Are there other ways by which we might be more effective? Almost without exception I was regarded as, at worst, antiprofessional, and at best, irrelevant.

There was a respite for me in the homes of people like Vera Watkins, Johnnie West, and Mertus Butler. I had my first piece of panfried cornbread in Mrs. Watkins' kitchen, sitting on a chair without a bottom. She would describe what she had to go through to get medical care for the children. I knew Mrs. Watkins didn't need to be "motivated" or "taught"; she just needed some means of obtaining health care without having to expend heroic amounts of effort to do so.

Johnnie and Mertus said essentially the same thing. They were younger. They had dreams that spilled out of them—and a lifetime to do something about those dreams. Health was not just prenatal care, it touched the wholeness of their lives.

I had stopped trying to teach the meaning of health. I listened. I took notes after talking with women like Mrs. Watkins and Johnnie and Mertus, and sixty others. I tabulated the mechanical problems they would mention about getting traditional kinds of health services—time, transportation, baby sitters. I asked them what would make it easier for them.

At the same time, through graduate work in sociology and anthropology in night school, I made a thorough ecological-demographic study of the neighborhood which, as I described it in my diary, "amounts to 105 pages, $130, twelve pounds of flesh, and less readily measurable costs. . . ." The statistics only confirmed what I had learned in people's homes and through the neighborhood groups. The only question then to ask was "So what?"

In response to my own question, I went to the director of the VNA, with a reminder of the promise I'd been given a year before. After two hours of questioning me, she asked for something in writing.

So I put on paper what women had told me in their homes, what the block clubs had been saying, and my own thoughts about what could be done. I clothed the proposal respectably with the data from my study and with the professional jargon in which I still believed. Only three or four pages long and asking for $15,000, it was the first of many drafts of what became the Maternity Satellite Project and then the Mom and Tots Center.

The modest proposal was still traditional in focus: it emphasized the prenatal period rather than the whole of life. This was done partly to gain the VNA's support and to have a traditional health rationale for seeking funds and partly because my own focus was still narrow. I saw day care, for example, as primarily a way to enable mothers to obtain "better prenatal care."

The project draft, with its tables and maps, implied my rational approach to change: if you just show people the facts you can convince them to do something about them. Today it is clear that neither the "facts" of the Kerner Report nor the smell of burning cities seem sufficient to move the nation toward healthful change.

The proposal called for consulting with professional specialists in community organization and child day care, which in the following months I did. It promised to involve neighborhood people, two of whom were Elma Hill and Mrs. Queen.

Up to this time I persisted in my faith in the basic soundness of the system of health and welfare agencies, of our social and political institutions. Even though the urban world as I knew it was not healthful and was not growing toward wholeness, I believed change could be realized through the existing agencies and organizations. We might have to wait awhile, but if we gathered our intellectual weaponry we could convince the decision-makers to allow us to work toward improving people's lives.

Certain events, both social and personal, following the spring of 1964 began to reshape me.

The quest for funds for the project gave me my first gut-awareness of bureaucratic complexities. My diary reflects my initial confusion; the meetings were "muddled"; they became "struggles." In the year that followed, I wrote, "There are an interminable number of steps. . . . It's very discouraging. . . . There are endless channels and detours. . . . I was told today not to go so fast. . . . I was cautioned about observing protocol. . . ." Finally, in the spring of 1965, money was promised under the medical wing of the Detroit poverty program.

At about this time, the Civil Rights movement was taking on a sense of urgency. Friends of mine, long-established professional people, now disillusioned, and increasingly fringe-members in their own professions, met to discuss what needed to be done. They were also among the supporters of the Northern Student Movement and ACME, which was then being organized. At that weekend enclave isolated from the city, ideas crashed against the walls and echoed in my head. I wrote, "My own thinking is forced to grow and to include more direct involvement in civil rights. . . ."

My friends arranged the meeting for me with Wilson Brown, the chairman of ACME at the storefront headquarters on Kercheval. They had described me to him previously as "a nurse who can lose her job if this thing (the 'Maternity Satellite Center') doesn't work." With that kind of introduction, before the advent of black power, our first discussion was conciliatory. I was excited by the prospects.

When two weeks later I returned and realized that Wilson and his cochairman had not read the project proposal, I felt for the first time a conflict which was to be repeated again and again, a conflict which was probably unresolvable. I could understand why they would not jump at the chance to read a proposal I had brought, particularly since the recent events in Selma had diverted their attention to more immediate problems. And I was unknown to them, a white professional. Besides, the paper was dull and stiff reading, even though, as proposals go, it was considered well written by my colleagues. But I knew that if I did not obtain ACME's criticisms and ideas soon, it would be difficult to change the project since the VNA was daily expecting to receive approval for funds and begin the implementation. At the same time, if they did not rise to my expectations—which were based on a romantic ideal of the downtrodden-but-forever-dynamic-and-struggling-black-freedom-fighter—my own administration might become critical of ACME's involvement in the project at all. In other words I wanted ACME to adapt to the system imposed upon me.

They did not adapt; not with any blatant refusal; they just did not adapt. And, without their knowing it, they were quite right. In effect, they were forcing me to implement one of the stated aims of the project, which was to find ways for health professionals and health care services to adapt to *them*.

In order to deal with this conflict, I began to learn to talk more pointedly to them, to describe the constraints placed upon me by TAP and the VNA. I reminded them how they were always complaining that no one ever asked them about the programs being designed for them; and, I said, I agreed with them and was trying as best I could under the circumstances to let them have something to say about what was going to happen in their neighborhood. If they wanted to let it go now, they'd better not complain later.

ACME responded with more feeling then, especially its

younger women, since the project was more ostensibly related to their interests.

The Protest March against the incident in Selma, Alabama, and the Freedom Train to Washington, D.C., two days later, were my first experiences in public demonstrations, conservative as they were.

The Freedom March did not move Congress to pass a strong Civil Rights Act in 1965, but it measurably altered my commitment; demonstrations may indeed alter the people involved in them more immediately than the circumstances at which they are aimed. I wrote in my diary, "Will my life take a drastic change? . . . I find myself a part of a movement (hardly a movement) rather a vision of a new world where men are whole and free to live responsibly. I suppose I have long believed in this vision, but now I am inextricably bound to it, or by it. . . ." Some of the personal decisions I had made I could see were not going to lead me in the direction I now wanted to go, and so I broke my wedding engagement. But I also knew, as I wrote to myself, "People who cannot risk involvement with people ought to acknowledge that they are sick. . . ."

And then word came that there was to be no money for the Maternity Satellite Project.

I had to face the ACME women. How could they see me as anything other than another member of the Establishment who had come to them with promises, now broken? All I could do was tell them what had happened, insofar as I understood it. They did not direct their anger at me. They were perhaps more verbal and articulate than I'd ever heard them. I gave them no timetables, but only the single promise that I knew I could keep: that I would continue trying to find a way to create the day-care program they now wanted, and then I'd return.

Behind my stoic demeanor was what I wrote in my diary, "There is no money for the project. I am at a loss to explain or describe how I feel. In a sense I am lost. . . . Perhaps I'm sorry for myself, tired, confused, . . . directionless; numb. I'm sure I must be angry. . . ."

The VNA accepted TAP's assurance that funding would be possible within two months and its recommendation that we go ahead and "mobilize" the people in the neighborhood. But I was skeptical and told my superiors that, judging from what I now knew about certain social and political circumstances locally and nationally, the project could not possibly be ready before the following Spring and could not be funded before January, 1966. Although events later confirmed my hunches, that did not assuage my feelings or improve my relationships to my superiors in the VNA. Having voiced my views, I felt I had been, as I wrote in my diary, "neatly and thoroughly cut down—gently, but firmly and thoroughly. . . ."

Months of silence followed, within the VNA agency and with neighborhood people, after I had visited each one to try to explain what had happened.

It was a painful silence, but the sounds of my own struggle thundered in me. I wrote in those months what I did not forget as I worked with people when the project later began, "How does one stop being afraid of one's feelings? . . . I'm being torn in two, pulled toward another world: the challenge to open the unlocked door, or to turn and run as I have before. But today I felt powerless to open the door; my hand shakes as I reach out for the handle, but then it drops. I don't know how to open it, much less know what's on the other side. . . . My life is a wound that I keep rubbing with salt. . . . What a fearsome awareness, to know that you are not communicating where you thought you had. . . . Tonight I played the piano for the first time in months and months; perhaps I'll learn again. . . . I'm learning that feeling intensely and feeling deeply are two different things. . . . Anger doesn't kill, only hate does. . . . I feel like I'm being born. . . ." At the end of the year I wrote, "I chose again to live, and if I have to I'll keep on choosing. . . ."

Two weeks before the beginning of 1966, a telegram announced that the VNA would receive $39,000 from the Office of Economic Opportunity to administer the Maternity Satellite Project. As a project administered independently of the TAP organization, I knew that potentially it could move more quickly and be more flexible, although the job of acquiring a building and renovating and equipping it, which was to have been TAP's province, was now mine.

I was afraid to begin for many reasons. I had a greater awareness of the complexities and contradictions inherent in the health and funding agencies related to the project than I had had the year before, and I was more acutely aware of attitudes within my own organization, the VNA. At the same time, I was beginning to understand the meaning of health in its many-faceted social and personal dimensions. I knew that I could not work with other people without wanting for them what I was learning about wholeness and without wanting to learn from them what I did not know.

So my goals and consequently those of the project were more broad and the means less simple, less direct, less predictable. I knew I would have to feel my way. I knew that I had to try to work with militant black people, even though their recent commitment to a black power stance would make this more difficult to do. I knew that trying to involve *only* militant people would isolate the project from the majority of nonmilitant Negroes, so these would be a part of the project too. Moreover, I no longer believed I could predict how the VNA would react to the direction which the project might take.

Finally, I knew that if the project did not really involve the people in the neighborhood, if it did not become what they wanted, then it would be a failure, whether or not it lasted. In any case, I could no longer go back to what I had known as community health nursing. My personal failure would be only in not *trying* to make the project a venture where wholeness was possible; not to *achieve* that goal would not be a failure.

So I began.

This time I first sought a meeting with the new chairman of ACME, Luke Pride. We could talk as intellectual peers. In private the differences in our skin color did not seem to matter; discussion flowed readily. The philosophical position which we shared was that people need the opportunity to find themselves, to develop their identity, personally and socially. From there, however, the differences began.

My skin disqualified the project from any real commitment he could offer it. He would not intentionally impede it, and he could even go along with it insofar as it did not jeopardize his leadership of ACME now that it was committed to black power. But when ACME members were present, which was most of the time, he used me as a symbol of the white authority figure. It was as though he were showing the young men and women of ACME how to deal with the white Establishment, how not to let it control them anymore, how to intimidate it; and then he would let them practice their lessons, so to speak, on me. And, the appointments they did not keep, the unanswered doorbells, the delays, were a way of dealing with "whitey," of reacting to a stereotype, in the manner that they had experienced all their lives by the white world.

In order for me to tolerate being reduced, though voluntarily, to an impotent stereotype, I had to keep reminding myself why it was happening. Why militant people were essential to the formation of the project. Why they were militant. Why they were responding to me as whitey. At that point, I did not allow myself the luxury of reacting in anger.

The few friends to whom I described some of these incidents, even those who accepted that black militancy was justified and necessary, urged me to avoid ACME. So I did not discuss these encounters with anyone, or those feelings which a person has when his best intentions are suspect, his valued thoughts and efforts belittled, his purposes scorned, his offers rejected, his self regarded as nonsignificant.

I was never certain that a vital link would be possible between the project and black power people, but I was always certain that I had to try to forge one. Yet I could sense that the time left to work at this, the days of toleration, were running out, both in terms of my psychological capacity and their ideological commitment.

In spite of all this, amid the gravity of the issues there was an excitement that was vitalizing, quite in contrast to the disillusioning and stifling interagency meetings in which I was concurrently engaged so as to attend to the funding paperwork and organizational relationships connected with the project.

So much for some of the events leading up to the meeting which occurred the last night in January, 1966. There is a significance both to those who were and were not present at it. Mrs.

Queen, who would have had an important role in the project if it had begun a year earlier, did not come. By electing to go back to school for a teaching certificate, she had chosen another means of making life better; her moderating influence was therefore absent.

Elma Hill too was absent. She was a friend of mine who would have been a volunteer. But in 1966 she was disqualified from working *at the Center* because of her category of affluent white person. However, she and her husband fulfilled a critical behind-the-scenes role for the Center later on in the political and financial struggles which ensued. Elma Hill accepted this limitation (which I would not have imposed the year before) because of her understanding, growing as mine was growing, of the meaning of people working significantly on their own behalf.

To be significant in an undertaking means that if you do not do your part, the job cannot get done. To be significant in a venture means to be essential to the whole. The variety of ideological and personality types in the Kercheval area had to be the essential contributors to the project, and the meeting on January 31 brought together many of those types.

It was very difficult for me to decline offers of volunteer help from friends and acquaintances, from other nurses and students. It was difficult to explain that if they and I were to put the project together, it would turn out to be *ours*. The project, if it was to be, was to belong to the people it was intended to serve, so *they* had to struggle to shape it and I with them for a while. *Then* it would be theirs. And when it was formed, I too would go.

It was difficult, too, for me to hear directly or indirectly that I did not value the contributions of my colleagues, that I did not want any help. That, of course, was not so; it was not that my insides did not sometimes cry out for softness and understanding. But the support, the encouragement I needed was not the kind of help my colleagues wanted to offer the project.

I was not able at that time to make clear that there is indeed an essential role for the concerned white affluent person in making whole our ghettoized cities. But it is a subtle role, often a nonvisible role. It is trying to do what black people cannot or will not do under any given circumstances until they are able or willing to do it. It is, therefore, a changing and a receding role, one that must persist until white and black stand facing each other as social equals, talking out and if necessary arguing out their differences without feeling unduly guilty or enraged.

On the night of January 31, I saw the women who gathered for the meeting and what they represented in a new way. Symbolically enough, they had divided themselves, the nonmilitants on one side, the ACME women on the other side, and I was left dividing the circle at the rim. Many had never met before. Their conversation was soon boisterous.

As I watched and listened, I realized that not only was there no such being as "the Negro," there were neither "militant" and "nonmilitant" black people, nor "middle-class-oriented" and "lower-class-oriented" people. If these are legitimately descriptive terms, then they refer to intertwining threads and not pigeonholes.

These women had experienced different facets of a Negro culture in a white society. They could laugh readily at problems common to all of them. I almost laughed, not so much at their jokes, as in thinking that these were the "lethargic," "unmotivated" people who are described in the reports of health and welfare workers. Nor were these "poor" people, whatever their income. They were rich in vitality and in an eagerness for a way that was better than what they had known.

The notion of a day-care program seemed to represent to them, in their commonalities and differences, a facet of "a way that was better."

I did not laugh at their jokes, for I finally saw that I was not one of them. I could not feel what they felt as they felt it, for I had not experienced it. And I did not have to, in order to work with them in the struggle toward wholeness. I was an "outsider," and could not pretend otherwise so long as we were all constrained to live in a racist world.

They were going to teach me, unwittingly, to see them not just as idealized symbols of the tragedy for which my white world was to blame, but as individuals unique in their subculture as I was in mine; and as individuals, too, sharing with me the physical, sensual, existential qualities common to all human beings. We would ultimately both lose and retain our categories, with comfort. But not yet.

That the name of the project was changed that night from Maternity Satellite Center to the Mom and Tots Center represented the shift which had been going on for more than a year, socially, ideologically, personally. The former name was professionally inspired, limited in focus, and placed the project ancillary to a hospital facility. The new name was at least as broad as the interests of these women, and it *centered* the project in their neighborhood. It marked the end of a long and painful first phase in the development of the Center, one which had sought and found a sufficient cohesion of ideas and aims, people and money to permit the next phase, a phase therefore as essential to its unfolding as those which followed.

II
Formation
of
a Matrix

Any real change implies the break-up of the world as one has always known it, the loss of all that gave one an identity, the end of safety.

JAMES BALDWIN
from *Nobody Knows My Name*

To compose a form through which life may unfold, a form which has potential for wholeness, requires the dynamic of diverse elements, the apparently irregular, the seemingly divergent. Such a form lacks the security of predictable behavior, but offers the possibility of newness.

The hiring policy for the Mom and Tots Center amounted to first come, first served, and no questions asked.

There was Ada Dixon, age forty-two, who lived with Mrs. Jefferson and her three children. She would quit her job as a hospital ward clerk to become secretary for the Center. "I'm very particular about my work. I don't like to make mistakes," she said. Mertus Butler had observed, "You won't find a better friend, if you can get her on your side."

Mrs. Jefferson wanted to work as a volunteer with young girls. Her own were nine and six. She would continue her job in a hospital operating room.

There was Felecia Thomas, a neighbor of Mertus. Her ideas rambled about with the same undisciplined ease that she seemed to have in tending to housekeeping. She lived with "Mother" and her sons Darrell, four, and Danny, eight months. Her husband Bernard was in the Air Force. Felecia said it was "hard to talk to them walls all day. The Mom and Tots Center sounds like something I could really be interested in!" She thought she'd like to cook, although Mother had done most of it at home; but she'd read up on protein and iron and work out some menus for the children. She'd try not to be a bother; she would talk to Mertus some more.

And there was nineteen-year-old Hank Edwards. ACME's Luke Pride had asked whether the Center could find work for him. Hank talked and thought and moved slowly. He had cerebral palsy. Because his muscles were contracted, he was forced to walk in a squat position. But he could shuffle up and down steps, and use his hands somewhat, and his heart. He was hired to do some maintenance work (everyone else knew they would have to help, too). "I'll do my very best," he said with difficulty. When he wasn't across the street sitting in

A C M E's window watching the Center, he was going about his chores or selling newspapers downtown.

Johnnie West also joined the staff. Her job was to think about what the women might like to have in a prenatal clinic. She had recently had a baby herself, so she could draw on her own experience. What would they enjoy most? What would she have wanted when she was pregnant?

And Mertus, who was to lead the day-care program, was busy reading, visiting, advising, and pestering her friends. She talked on and on about how they would give the children "new experiences," "enhance their creativity," and "involve their parents." There would be field trips, swings and slides, a piano, puppet shows and plays, and even motion pictures. Her description included no notion as to *how* these things might come about.

And Mrs. Watkins. She would work in the day-care program—mothering the children. "I just know they all going to find something wrong with me so's I can't work," she said almost every step of the way. "They" did not find anything in anyone that was not remediable in one way or another. Mrs. Watkins began her first job, though it might have been a little hard for her to believe, "Why you all going through such a bother for me?" . . .

The Kercheval storefront and second-floor apartment which were to become The Mom and Tots Center gradually changed in appearance.

When the necessary building permits were requested of various city bureaus, the response was the same: It sounds like a good program, but why can't you locate in a better neighborhood? But the approvals were granted.

Pete Collins Jackson worked in his own style: making phone contacts after 11 P.M.; supervising his subcontractors late into the night—plumber, electrician, carpenters, painters from the neighborhood; asking for advances of $500 to $900 in order to buy materials; controlling his anger at overhearing "nigger!" and other epithets from the squat Macedonian landlady, Rilka Vasiloff. She kept a close watch on her property, one of ten storefronts. He promised the tile would be laid no later than February 25.

ACME agreed to move in a truck load of clinic furniture donated by World Medical Relief. WMR, at their West Side warehouse, had the equipment ready to be picked up on February 25. A truck was rented.

But on February 25 the tile had not been laid. And Luke, who was to drive the truck, said an emergency had come up: as bondsman he had to go with one of his boys to court.

The ACME storefront got into motion. Who could drive the truck? Who could carry the furniture? Chester had lost his chauffeur's license. James was working today.

Luke whispered to Larry. Larry said he'd help carry the furniture. Willy "the Kercheval Pimp" came in; he'd work too.

Carter arrived with Abraham, the defendant. After more discussion on transporting the "goods" interspersed with questions about what was going to go on at the Mom and Tots Center, Abraham said, "Hey man, nobody's thinking about me!"

Finally, Carter suggested renting a trailer. He could pull it with his big Oldsmobile.

Two trailer-loads of furniture were on the sidewalk in front of Mom and Tots by 2:30 that afternoon. Carter had to leave quickly to get to work. Luke came over, and with Roosevelt and Bill who were walking past, carried it to the second floor and piled it all in two rooms, to leave space for the tile to be laid.

ACME often came to the rescue of Mom and Tots in the next few weeks, moving a refrigerator, a piano, hammering open almost with glee the iron gates which Rilka Vasiloff had locked around the Center (these were removed before the Center opened April 1).

The encounters were not always pleasant, especially when feelings were aroused about being hired by a white outsider; no amount of money was acceptable. "Listen, Little Moma, I don't want no chump change." Or when there was talk about the white power structure; one leader in the Black Freedom Now Party concluded his argument with "You ought to get out. A Black person ought to be where you are."

Privately, Luke would say in a quiet tone that ACME was not going to be able to reach the older women with children; that Mom and Tots could get to them, and to people in the block clubs and churches; that the services would be good, but would not change people's lives. Mom and Tots should expect to be frustrated if it wanted to reach the kind of women who belonged to ACME, women whose priorities were "non-middle class"; who fought the system and who needed to find a way to express their pride in being black.

In front of ACME members, Luke would allow heated exchanges and then at their peak end them abruptly with "O.K. Cool it!"

Renovations progressed, transforming the storefront into the Mom and Tots Center. It then became a natural setting for comfortable interchange among the people who would work there, as they went about the tasks of interior decorating.

Ada Dixon and Mrs. Jefferson were concerned about getting just the right kind of curtains for the Center. At the suggestion of getting together with some of the ACME women to make them, Ada said "Why do we have to include them, when they don't cooperate? They won't do the job as good as we can anyway." And Mertus thought that they didn't have "ideas like we have." They stood firm on curtain-making, but agreed to allow ACME women to come to a chair-painting session on the next Monday evening. They would bring coffee.

They telephoned Jeannie, who agreed to come to the meeting. She would contact other ACME women.

That Monday, Ada, Mrs. Jefferson and her three children arrived at the Center and began the painting. Vera Watkins joined them after she had prepared her 4 o'clock supper for her family. Then came Felecia playing pranks with Mertus. Mertus joked about seeing "the boss" work. Ada did not stay for the evening's discussion, "I been here all day." And Mrs. Jefferson had to take the children for their music lessons.

No one came from ACME.

Ada did not have bus fare to get to the next evening work session. She waited for Mertus who was bringing her daughter, preschooler Kay; then they were delayed with a flat tire.

Mrs. Watkins came with Deneen. Felecia brought Darrell. "Do you think I'm too silly?" she asked. "Some people say I am. I could be real formal if you want; but I'd rather just be me."

Ada was perturbed with the children running around. With a claw hammer she tore off an old hinge from the window sill, chipping the new paint. Then she rewashed the windows Mertus had just finished. "Hey, those windows were just washed." "*Were* they?" Later, she raised her hammer in mock threat over a minor incident.

The discussion at coffee break that night centered on family planning. Ada went on with her work and did not join it.

The next day in her home, Ada had much to say, given the opportunity. She was impatient that the Center was not opening yet; here it was the middle of March. . . . The work was poorly organized; it was not neat. . . . Then there were Mertus' "crazy ideas" to put up with, and the kids dirtying the woodwork. . . . And "You remind me of a white woman I knew in Mississippi eighteen years ago. I hated her . . ." And "ACME is Black Nationalist—I don't want no part of them . . ." She was only joking when she raised that hammer. . . . Sometimes she gets "despondent" when she isn't busy; she has "bad nerves"; and sometimes she gets migraines. Sometimes she won't talk to people when she's "peeved." Yes, a doctor has given her pills to help her relax.

Ada listened when she heard that Mom and Tots had to try to reach as many people in the neighborhood as possible, including ACME, even if that seemed hopeless. The people at Mom and Tots had to try to trust each other, and work together like a team, and talk to each other when there was doubt or anger, so that they wouldn't have to raise hammers to each other.

"I ain't never thought about it that way before," she said. "Maybe I can try."

There was some typing she could do for the Center. She'd get busy on that.

Mertus and Felecia, Mrs. Jefferson, and the others were looking for bargains in day-care equipment, wholesale food, kitchen utensils. The children in the neighborhood volunteered for odd jobs and errands or came "just to watch" during their lunch period. One of the first to try to discover what the Center was all about was little Tommie Sanderson, an eight-year-old brother of one of Luke's boys. Tommie was one of ten children, and he got little attention at home. His teachers called him incorrigible and overactive and often put him out of school. He regularly left his finger marks on the Center walls—which annoyed some of the staff, who just didn't like him to "hang around."

The major renovations were completed. But the workmen were complaining that their checks from Pete Collins Jackson had bounced. "I sure hope this place works out for you all," said Eddie, the painter. "And I sure hope I get my money." He eventually tried to take his fee from Pete Collins Jackson directly, and wound up in jail on an assault and battery charge.

The electrician and carpenter took their case to court. They eventually got some of their money, but the Internal Revenue Service had prior claim to the unpaid balance of Pete Collins alias Jackson's $4000 contract with the VNA.

It was time for the first official meeting of the Mom and Tots "staff"—the new label sounded strange and unfamiliar. The meeting place was upstairs in the clinic unit, newly painted in blues, and green, and yellow.

Hank Edwards wandered through the examining rooms, once bedrooms, the desk area, the kitchen, and crib room, stroking the walls almost as though they were alive.

Ada Dixon was in a red dress instead of her usual skirt and

sweater. She was heartily complimented on her printed cafe curtains that covered the bay window in the reception and coffee area, and the striped curtains decorating the other rooms. She spoke of the importance of working together at Mom and Tots.

The staff heard again how the Center was going to try to respond to all kinds of people in the neighborhood, including ACME; how they needed to talk frankly with each other—not just wait until weekly staff meetings. Questions, ideas, problems had to be talked about when they occurred. Just because a thing had been done one way did not mean it could not be changed. Just because a thing had never been done before did not mean it could not be tried. Whatever rules Mom and Tots would set up would apply to everyone there—workers, visitors, patients, children, adults.

Mrs. Watkins offered many nods and "Amens." Her only verbal response was in reference to ACME, "That don't mean we got to go on no protest marches!"

Hank said that there were some people at ACME who would dislike certain people no matter what color they were.

Mertus thought that ACME could not be trusted.

And Mrs. Jefferson implied that anyone willing to listen to ACME could not be trusted either. They (Mrs. Jefferson and her friends) could "listen to our own kind" better than anyone else.

Everyone agreed that the Mom and Tots workers were best able to listen for and understand what people in their neighborhood wanted most, and they could relay this to the powers that be. They would be polite to *anyone* that came into the Center, but they sure wouldn't go across the street to ACME.

Johnnie, holding Grace on her lap, wanted to talk about the preschoolers. She said how important it was to give a lot of personal attention to every child.

Mertus described how every child would have his name emphasized, he would be greeted individually, his snapshot would be taken, his drawings would be labeled on the ceiling-high burlap bulletin boards downstairs. She tried to explain the difference between closed- and open-ended questions and why the staff should try to be "open-ended": to ask questions which couldn't be answered with a simple yes or no. The technique was new to her, too.

"I have a question," said Felecia. "What are we going to do about the bathrooms in day care? I mean, what are we going to teach the children about keeping the doors closed? And what if there's two of them in there together? I mean, a boy and a girl"?

"Of course them doors ought to be shut! And one child in there at a time," Ada said definitively.

"Well I don't think it would hurt the children if the doors were open," Johnnie offered.

If the children were to grow up to be proud and happy about what they are, wasn't the fact that they were male or female something to be happy and proud of too?

Ada groaned in exasperation.

Mertus tentatively concluded that they could let the children do whatever they wanted about the bathroom door.

Mrs. Watkins cast a sidewise glance.

"I was thinking of getting some symphony music for the children," Mertus continued.

"You mean we can't have something with some Soul?" Felecia said.

Then came a discussion on which kind of music was better.

Had anyone ever heard bagpipes? French folk tunes? Spanish guitars? Russian music? Oriental instruments? Perhaps the children could hear these too. Then they could decide for themselves what they liked best.

Mertus was agreeable. The others were dubious.

She then explained that a consultant, Mr. Hughes, had been asked to help them in the day-care program about once a week. She told them that a consultant was someone they could listen to, but that they didn't have to do what he said.

Mr. Hughes was a teacher and writer, blond and blue-eyed, who had lived in a Philadelphia ghetto. His efforts to broaden the staff's perceptions of their environment sometimes seemed to go too far, as when he tried to have them appreciate the aesthetics of the stones from the alley, the flies, the dandelions.

"Hell," said Ada, "What do I want to appreciate all that junk for?"

"I sure don't want my kids playing with that stuff," said Mrs. Watkins.

The younger women were slightly more receptive, though skeptical.

The finishing touches were being added as Mom and Tots prepared to open its doors officially.

The staff had gotten its physical examinations, x rays, immunizations, and food-handler's cards. A number of problems were identified and taken care of:

Felecia's breast biopsy was negative.

Mrs. Watkins' anemia was under treatment.

Mertus began using birth control pills.

Ada Dixon had new eyeglasses.

Plans were made for Hank to undergo long-term treatment at a rehabilitation center in early summer.

And all their children were examined and treated as necessary, which was frequently.

Mrs. George, a Negro practical nurse, who wanted to "adopt all the children at Mom and Tots," provided transportation to the array of clinics needed by the staff. And she offered her services to the Center "any time of the day (she worked at night) for as long as you need me."

Mertus prepared a "Daily Plan for Day Care," typewritten, and presented it, along with Mr. Hughes, to the others.

```
10:30   ARRIVAL and FREE PLAY
            (Children each should be greeted
        warmly and encouraged to play with
        the play material in the center.
        During this time the aides will take
        children individually to the bath-
        room and see to the child brushing
        his teeth. Be sure always to listen
        to the children; what the children
        say is important.)
```

```
11:15   STORY TIME
            (Read a story that you are well
            familiar with; be able to tell it
            by memory almost. Allow the children
            to ask questions freely; also allow
            them to add to the story with their
            own imagination or to create a new
            story.)

11:30   QUIET TIME (Song time and music time)

12:00   LUNCH

12:30   CRAFT TIME: SCIENCE TIME:
        EXCURSION TIME

 1:30   Parents pick up children
```

Felecia tried to study some menus prepared by a retired Irish cook. She had not become confident enough to work out her own menus as required by the day-care licensing bureau.

Johnnie discussed the prenatal clinic with a young VNA nurse, Mrs. Carol Howard: white, bright, dedicated to taking care of people, she would work at Mom and Tots two days a week, especially in the prenatal program.

Ada Dixon confidently accepted the task of planning an Open House for April 1. Mertus said Mrs. Jefferson would help if she were asked. She was—and she did.

Fliers announcing "You are cordially invited to an Open House . . ." went to neighborhood churches, storefronts, and block clubs. Tommie Sanderson and his little friends passed them up and down their streets.

On April 1 the day-care area was ready for visitors. Short pink, white, and green bamboo curtains framed the storefront windows. Spring flowers, cookies, and coffee were on the counter which divided the kitchen from the play area. Mertus and Felecia had climbed up on ladders to fill the bulletin boards; at the top was their reminder: "Children Are Important: Talk To Them, Listen To Them, Play With Them, Love Them."

The sky was dark. It was raining. By 3 o'clock Ada's Guest Book showed only nine visitors, and seven of them were from the District Office of the VNA.

But after school, the children came. Then a neighbor of Mrs. Watkins. Then Mrs. Patterson, who went back home to get her pregnant cousin. Then Mrs. Crockett and her three children. And Mrs. Ward, who was afraid she was pregnant. And Mrs. Steel. Veronica Shoemaker, age seven, came in for a cookie and pulled her mother in. The leader in the Freedom Now Party came too, and said that Mom and Tots should be working with ACME since they were both working for the same thing. . . . The open house was a success.

When she thought no one was looking, Mertus took Tommie Sanderson and pushed him out the back door.

To
form
a matrix

consisting of a building complex
and staff of workers which would generate a sense of life was for
me a task without blueprint. I knew only that no matrix could
generate life if it were not alive, and that vitality was not a quantity to be added after the matrix was formed. It would be present
only if allowed expression and growth in the formative process.

At the outset I learned that there were implications to
every choice that I made—and to whether or not I allowed others
to make choices. Each choice would move the project, however
imperceptibly, either closer to or farther from its focus toward
wholeness.

I tried to be aware of the implications to my choices,
whether it was deciding if neighborhood children should be allowed in the Center, or where to look for a contractor, or how the
furniture should be moved, or what the qualifications of the staff
should be, or who should make the window curtains.

School children allowed in the storefront meant, at the
least, finger prints and cooky crumbs. But doors closed to them
meant the cutting off of a potential source of life and intercourse

49

with the neighborhood. So the building remained open to them, except when particular programs were in session—contrary to Ada's wishes.

Seeking a contractor from the neighborhood obviously carried more risk than dealing with a well-known firm. But hiring neighborhood tradesmen meant that poverty program funds for building renovations would be going into the ghetto as the Congressional legislation intended, and not to an affluent contracting firm. Because we were under pressure to begin immediately (the funds were granted on a year to year basis only), and because there were a limited number of available contractors in the neighborhood, Pete Collins Jackson had to be the one, in spite of his work style, and much to the dismay of my superiors. Although it would have been preferable to avoid the legal entanglements which followed, the Center gained by the experience in several ways: most of the work was done more quickly than a large firm could have done it; it was another thread connecting the Center to ACME and eventually to Pete Collins Jackson's sons, who were avowed militant Black Nationalists; and it communicated in a concrete way the intentions of the Center to both use the resources of the neighborhood as well as to invest its resources there.

The experience also gave me another view of someone I might otherwise regard as simply a crooked contractor. I cannot label Pete Jackson so glibly now. I saw the bare floors and walls of his house and the thin clothes on his children, of whom there were at least six. I know he had a construction job during the day, collected and sold used parts, and peddled fruit in the summertime. Under other circumstances he might be called "enterprising," "a shrewd businessman," a "hardworking family man." But he didn't cover his checks fast enough.

Moving furniture and equipment to the Center was itself an unforeseen problem, because the health institution which had agreed to provide these in 1965 decided against doing so in 1966. Thus, the Center, without budgeted funds, had to seek donated equipment and furnishings. Again, this was an opportunity to relate to ACME. ACME was a source of unemployed men who could gain by the fee for moving. Hiring a moving company would divert money out of the area as well as avoid the complications which would almost inevitably occur with ACME. So, contrary to the advice of my superiors in the VNA, ACME did the moving. I was in the back seat of Carter's Oldsmobile as five ACME men carted two loads of equipment back and forth across the city. I saw them in a different way than I had before. I saw men who worried about their little sisters and about their women, who got lost in traffic, who complained about the cold, and enjoyed warmth and comfort; men who talked softly and cared about themselves and about those they loved.

And what qualifications ought the staff of the Center to have? They were experts in seeing life from the perspective of the ghetto and so could help mold the Center into a setting that could be home to the ghetto dweller. That they accepted the idea of a Mom and Tots Center enough to want to work with it was qualification enough. That they knew there was no "how to do it" but were willing to find a way was what the Center needed. Their history—employment, marital, court—would not disqualify them; it was not asked about.

After months of working with them I saw another aspect of the tragedy of the ghetto: there must be so many vibrant people working there, unknown to us, perhaps unknown to themselves; undiscovered wealth because they do not meet certain "qualifications."

It was a disparate group of individuals that began. I was fascinated by the possibilities of a new integration of personal qualities, as well as frightened by the likelihood of collapse. In the beginning collapse seemed the more imminent. The staff's limitations were often more evident than their positive strengths: Ada's compulsive orderliness; Mertus' planlessness; Felecia's childishness; Mrs. Watkins' reluctance to engage in certain activities, such as reading to the children, because she had little formal education. But because I had known some of them in their homes for months or years, and had listened to them under other circumstances, I felt I knew their potential. How to deal with their inner conflicts was another matter. My own preference would have been to talk with them about themselves directly. But I had no way of knowing how articulate they were about themselves, how self-aware, or how much of an intrusion they might regard my speaking to them about themselves. I did not know how much of a barrier my skin color would be or my official position as an authority figure.

But, for several reasons, talking could not be left to chance; the problem of how people ought to face each other could not be avoided. The staff members needed to become more articulate: to discover their own ideas and to put those ideas into action. There were also too many areas of potential conflict and misunderstanding—in terms of race, social background and values—for these differences not to be expressed, if not understood. In other words, talking was a part of the meaning of health.

I chose the afternoon and evening work sessions at the Center, which were ostensibly intended to accomplish the interior decorating, as the setting to expose ideas and feelings before the group. Usually, the concreteness of the circumstances, the fact that people were busy with their hands, that we were all doing the same things, allowed both light and serious conversation, not too intense or too threatening. I often would wait until a coffee break and then elicit their reactions to a particular subject, for example, who should be allowed to obtain birth control at the center?

In time, as the opening of the Center approached, regular staff meetings were held where people were ready and able to engage in more direct and prolonged discussion. One subject which should not have been voiced directly and so early in the formation of the group involved confronting black people with the meaning of being black. This was done by Mr. Hughes, a white man, at one of two early staff meetings which he attended. While I could not have stated at that time why he should not have done this, I could feel the women bristle and freeze into silence and would therefore have shifted the discussion. But the damage was quickly done, as Mertus told me later that night. The women allied me with Mr. Hughes and became suspicious of my intentions as well as his. Although in the following nine months, he was able to repair some of the damage as he met with them every week or two, he made a couple of similar errors in judgment which ultimately ended his effectiveness. He would have been the first to say that they indeed determined who should be allowed to work with them.

I too paid for being identified with the assumption that white people can help black people attain their identity as black people, implying that we as white people have already gained our own. It is no more than a contemporary version of the white paternalism of a generation ago. Being involved in the Mom and Tots venture helped me put into words what only my insides told me in the beginning. It is in our equivalence as human beings that we help to define each other, not as people in one category molding people in another category.

In the two years which followed, having worked with the staff and seen them respond through two racial upheavals, one of the worst in the history of the United States, I know that it was not that they were not ready, as I then thought, to deal with their identity as black people, although I am sure that as individuals some were more and some less able to be articulate about themselves, but they were not willing to talk about it with white people. I saw this willingness change in time for many reasons: they had put me in the position of a learner rather than teacher; the racial unrest so dramatically expressed in the cities had put blackness on everyone's lips; changes at the Center were made to encourage them to be more explicit about blackness among themselves and their programs; and they may indeed have been less willing to deny to the white world that "black is beautiful," just as a few white people are becoming more willing to say that white is beautiful too, and that the two are not mutually exclusive.

But as with other changes that I saw, I could never be sure whether the "change" was due to an actual alteration or transformation in them, or to a change in me and my perceptions, or to their allowing me to see more of what was there all the while. Perhaps it was all of these.

The whole explosive issue of the expression of racial identity was quelled after I talked individually with Mertus and with Ada, each of whom then conveyed my intentions to the others. By the time of the first official staff meeting, the related issue of the Center's association with ACME women—whom the other women at least regarded as using shameful means of expressing their racial selves—was quietly settled also. In effect, they would accept ACME, but not take any initiative to draw it to the Center; I could if I wanted to. And *they*, the staff, not I, would interpret what other people in the neighborhood wanted, so that the Center could respond accordingly. Where I had seen the commonalities they shared with the ACME people at that meeting on January 31, I had not realized the intense antagonism that they also felt.[1] Perhaps the most basic common tie which they all had was their hostility to the white world, expressed in varying ways, some obvious, like ACME's, some subtle like my staff's.

I was immensely pleased that they felt free enough to express their anger in words at the staff meeting in deciding what would be done.

I never again raised these questions of race with them directly, although after a few months, I took steps to try to have them face themselves consciously and to shape the Center to encourage this for other people. But this I would try to do with any group of people with whom I worked, black or white.

In those first weeks and months I thought it unwise and unnecessary to engage in individual confrontations which might become too intense or threatening. However, I thought I had no choice but to talk very pointedly to Ada, because her hostility seemed so extreme, sometimes subtle, often overt; it was apparent in almost everything she did and said. I seriously questioned whether she might be too divisive a force in the Center. But I wanted to talk directly to her before making any decisions. So I went to her house. Because of the incident with the hammer, which had been raised at me, I was afraid.

I looked straight at her, and she responded in kind. She seemed to want a chance to talk. I could hear behind her words, although I did not know her history, that she had rather severe psychological problems under certain circumstances. In a sense, we are all psychological casualties of our life experiences; but I thought the Center ought to at least try to encompass as many fringe people as it could. Besides, Ada's assets were clearly present, if only the Center and she could focus on them.

That conversation, which lasted almost two hours, initiated a change in the basis of our relationship. I believed her when she said she would try to be aware of the effects of her behavior.

In time, after some structural changes at the Center, Ada became as intense in her thoroughness and loyalty to the Center as she had been hostile.

Because the staff were a part of the ghetto, they were encumbered with all of the mechanical problems which nonaffluent people perpetually face: very little cash, transportation and babysitting problems, erratic hours, little crises that become big ones when there are no ready means to deal with them. What made it hard for them to obtain health care also made it difficult for them to attend meetings at the Center. So provision was made for helping them get health care for their whole families; transportation and babysitting were a part of all the work sessions and meetings at the Center. And later a petty cash system was devised.

These arrangements were in effect before the Center opened; they served several purposes, in addition to meeting the immediate needs of the staff. Learning how to accommodate their own everyday problems provided useful experience, for in order to perform a family-centered service, the staff would have to take into account these same mechanical but crucial problems of daily living, obstacles as they are to so many endeavors. And the arrangements were a way of saying that although the Center was not going to be a health structure in the traditional sense, it recognized that the soul, the mind, the self, could not very readily find a way when the body was exhausted or in pain or discomfort.

I led the staff meetings in what amounted to an informal group dynamics fashion. They were often preceded by joking and by queries about what might be bothering the members personally, such as how was Mrs. Watkins' stiff knee, or was Kay still home from school with a cold, or what had Felecia heard from her husband in the Air Force? I was often able to cut some red tape for them with their family problems. Soon they expressed their concerns more readily and offered suggestions to each other. Increasingly, my leadership became less direct as they discussed problems related to the Center. Eventually, I would be more or less "sitting in."

Discussing the development and emphases of the day-care

program, as well as other programs, served the less obvious purpose of making visible their ideas and mine about the meaning of wholeness, how it is developed, and of what it consists.

They were very concerned that the children learn to speak well, and soon came to understand that language and ideas are developed when children are listened to, when they are not given answers in the questions that are asked them. (This was why I worked with Mertus on "open-ended" questions). Children come to know their intrinsic worth when their offerings are accepted because they are authentic. Realness is the criterion of acceptance, not someone's standard of taste. A child's name is the symbol of himself, and therefore it is special. Indirectly we were, of course, talking about ourselves.

The question about the closed bathroom door implied a whole conception of sexuality that connoted shame and restrictiveness. Judging from some of the responses to the idea of allowing an open door, I regarded the decision not to decide an accomplishment. It is hard to say which aspect of individual identity was more emotion-laden, the racial or sexual. The topic of sexuality itself was for a long time not raised directly by the staff, although it often appeared indirectly, as with the bathroom door problem. Again, I could not know whether their difficulty in discussing it, much less considering a broader conception of sexuality, was a reflection of the common American inarticulateness on the subject, or their own limited vocabulary or uncertainties about their own feelings, or a way to avoid perpetuating the stereotype which many white people hold of the black person as an oversexed being, with all the overtones of immorality that carries. And again, these were probably all factors. However, I was learning to proceed indirectly and with caution and, in time, had some success, at least in the area of verbal expression.

Whether discussing choices among music or food, styles of dress or decor, social or personal behavior, the pull was toward an either/or selection. For example, *either* symphonic music *or* Soul music, the preference often being the former during the first months of the Center; this seemed to represent a better way; it meant the way of life of the American middle class. In discussing these choices they talked as though there were two ways open to human development: the style of the white affluent and that of the black poor, and the former was the better.

I did not know how to tell them that they could legitimately aspire to the comforts and conveniences of affluence without derogating their own cultural style; that, in fact, their spontaneity and informality might enrich the lives of the more sophisticated.

Since the implications of their choices seemed to me so grave, I tried to broaden the range of possibilities from which they would choose, and to emphasize, but not too pointedly, that life did not have to be an either/or proposition;[2] at least our visions did not have to be divided that way. I trod cautiously, however, since I did not want to imply that being poor in economic terms was good or gratifying.

The central problem in the formation of an organization, even a small one, is said to be the coherent development of a core staff, a staff whose outlook reflects the basic philosophy of the organization.[3] Basic to the development of this group is the discussion of policy issues and the sharing of key experiences, especially internal conflicts and other crises.

This time-consuming phase seems to me even more important when, as in the case of the Center, the members of the group are drawn from divergent ways of life. I represented a facet of one subculture, and my staff varying facets of another subculture. Sharing a range of experiences together began the formation of a kind of new subculture—a new set of ways of doing—one unique and essential to the further development of the Center. Thus, the painting sessions contributed to our cohesion as a group, as well as made the storefront itself a product of the staff's hands and their aesthetic. This was why I sought to have everyone present at each session, and why I sought A C M E women as well. That A C M E women did not come was their own decision, although a disappointment to me.

The arguments and discussions over ideas and methods, the joking, even the subtle and overt expressions of hostility added to our fund of common ties. It was not necessary to think or feel alike about the same experiences, but only to have an opportunity to talk about them, to hear how others felt about them; in other words, to share the experience, not necessarily the response.

The *way* in which these experiences were shared as well as the *kinds* of experiences, served to communicate certain ideas, experientially as well as verbally. The staff learned the importance of talking and listening, of trying out suggestions and offering choices, of setting up rules and applying them equally; they would use these approaches as they in turn dealt with the families who came to the Center.

Attending to the facets of their own unfolding would help them understand its meaning as they worked with the people and programs in the Center, although the transfer was by no means automatic.

The tempo of the first day, the Open House, forecast the rhythm which the Center would take on, having a kind of reawakening in mid or late afternoon. This change in tone, consistent with the movement of the neighborhood, was very apparent at the Center, and predictable. It seemed to encompass something more than that children came home from school at 3:30, and men returned from or left for work then, though those factors were basic to it. The pace of life began slowly and late in the morning, revived in late afternoon, and was vibrant after dark, especially on warm nights. In seeking a harmony with the neighborhood, the Center, too, took on this tenor.

Such a rhythm, so different from the early morning bustle of a VNA district office, was cause for disappointment in the visitors who came from the district office. They said they had expected the whole neighborhood to be there; they were not to return for two years.

I saw no reason to expect a large crowd for the Open House, considering the rainy weather and the as yet unproved worth of the Center to the neighborhood. But I said none of this to my former coworkers; it would only have sounded like a rationalization to them. Instead, I listened, uncomfortably, to their fears for my failure. And it would indeed have been *my* failure in their eyes, as in their eyes it was *my* "clinic" (for more than a year they referred to the Center as a clinic, a term which I constantly corrected).

I watched the response of the people at the Center, especially the staff, to the few outsiders who came from time to time, such as my colleagues, or the Irish cook who came perhaps a half-dozen times, as long as the staff asked her. It was only after many months that I could see clearly how very different they appeared when a strange white person came in, presenting themselves with feigned ignorance, ineptness, or naiveté. I could not help but wonder what variant of themselves had existed or continued in their relations with me. I would never know.

This abrupt and apparent personality change was no less stark than the ways in which Mrs. Vasiloff, the landlady, treated Pete Collins Jackson when she was, and when she was not aware of my presence; or, later, the manner in which health professionals treated patients when they were and were not aware of being overheard.

The day of the Open House marked the completion of the physical matrix of the storefront, transformed as it was by as many hands if not hearts from the neighborhood as would respond. The staff had begun to be tied together by common efforts. And they had translated some of the ideas which were essential to the Center into the motto which Mertus and Felecia put on the wall, about talking, listening, playing, loving.

An idea, finding a link with ghetto life, had coalesced into a place. For myself, I found it hard to believe that the Center was now something that could be seen and touched, walked in and out of, lived in.

III
Discovering the Possible

To meld diversity, but maintain openness;
To foster stability, but remain vulnerable to new perspectives;
To allow repose, but maintain a pregnant attitude;
To face complexity, but maintain simplicity and directness.
This is the problem, the challenge,
Of a setting, a group, an individual
That would be whole.

On the Monday morning following the Open House Mertus, Felecia, and Mrs. Watkins were waiting to welcome mothers who came to enter their children in day care—sometimes, in their enthusiasm, giving answers to questions that weren't asked. Sometimes giving the answers in the questions they asked. Sometimes forgetting that a mother might need help in getting a medical check-up or "shots" for her preschooler, or forgetting that there were other people in the family who might need something the Center could offer, or not explaining clearly that payment was to be made in time, not money. Mothers were to spend one or two hours every other week in the day-care program instead of paying a fee.[1]

At the same time, the staff was sensitive to feelings in the women which they themselves shared.

After an older married couple left the Center, they said, "You shouldn't have talked about birth control in front of her husband, even if she did want it. Couldn't you see it embarrassed him?"

Looking out the window, they could see a rotund woman in distress. They invited her in and sat her down. She had just heard that her son, Steve Lewis, had been injured at school and taken to City hospital. But she had no phone and no carfare. They showed her to the phone, and she called the hospital and then a brother to drive her there.

The next day, Mrs. Lewis enrolled her preschooler Michael in day care. She became the first to volunteer her time and often remained longer than the expected two hours. "I just want to. I don't know nobody in the neighborhood."

During enrollment week as Mertus entered the first fifteen

children into day care, she raised many questions that took hours to resolve:

They were looking for pictures of parents and children to put up on the walls. She suggested they take them from *McCall's* instead of *Ebony*. "After all," she said, "It's up to the Negro to make the adjustment to the white world."

And they should have a half-hour of coffee time between their 9 A.M. to 3 P.M. work day.

They needed more games and blocks she said. Those little chairs were too expensive. She didn't like the newsprint for drawing. It took so long for the materials on order to arrive. She knew she was going to run out of chalk and paint.

And what about Felecia, now that she had enrolled her son Darrell in day care? When was she going to contribute her payment in time?

And, don't worry about how she would handle the first day when the program began next week. She'd do "something." . . .

The pictures on the walls came out of *Ebony*.

The staff took coffee breaks when they needed them.

A cash fund, replenished monthly, was devised for the Center, and distributed for each program:

Mertus (*day care*)	$10	
Felecia (*day-care food*)	55	(*on account at a local supermarket*)
Ada (*clerical*)	5	
Johnnie and Carol Howard, the nurse (*clinic supplies and children's clubs*)	25	
Mrs. Jefferson (*Girl's Club*)	5	
	$100	

Felecia contributed time during prenatal clinic or for other special events.

And the first day of day care was left to Mertus.

Early the next Monday morning, although delayed by a policeman who issued her a ticket for "disturbing the peace" with a defective carburetor, Mertus was at the Center, washing the floor for the first day-care session. Hank had not used "enough elbow grease" to satisfy her.

She greeted the children[2] as they came, introducing them to the blackboards and drawing boards that lined the lower walls, inviting them to the toys in the cupboards.

Mrs. Watkins just couldn't see how you could let children help themselves, since they "mess up the place." She and Felecia huddled behind the kitchen counter, serving coffee to mothers, preparing lunch—perhaps giving more time to the hot dogs, carrot sticks, and layers of fruit-filled jello than they needed. When they finally emerged from the kitchen, Felecia pleased herself and the children with animated reading from the story books. Mrs. Watkins was reluctant to try.

The food tasted good—the adults paid a quarter to lunch with the children. Tooth paste was a new taste for some. The weights and measurements were fairly accurate and fun besides. The snapshots turned out well and were soon displayed on the burlap boards.

And there was Tommie Sanderson, looking in the window. School children were not allowed in during day care.

During individual conversations at the Center or by late evening phone calls, Mertus reacted to her new position. She often felt out of breath, " 'cause the children won't sit still at story time." And Felecia and Mrs. Watkins didn't seem to understand that she was in charge. She had the hardest time getting them out of the kitchen. Mrs. Watkins didn't seem interested; she never said anything. . . . Then, Ada Dixon was upset when Mertus was late; Mertus admitted, "I just can't get organized in the morning, seems like; but I do try."

Perhaps it wasn't necessary for all the children to sit and listen to stories at the same time; and perhaps Felecia and Mrs. Watkins might venture out of the kitchen if they could do things they enjoyed doing. Could Mertus solicit their ideas and act upon their suggestions? Then they might accept her guidance more readily. And would being a little more organized help establish their confidence in her?

Mertus thought. She wanted a workshop, the three of them and Mr. Hughes. She wrote an outline. They could discuss the purposes of day care, practice some techniques, and talk about attitudes. They could each lead in certain areas: songs, bulletin boards, chalk talks, games, science, trips, crafts, stories, rhymes. . . . She eventually asked for a policy of "docking" late-comers. The staff agreed, but allowed for make-up time.

In June, not long after the eight-hour workshop had been held, Mertus glowed: Felecia was inventing puppet shows and chalk talks, and stimulating dramatic play. Mrs. Watkins was telling stories from pictures and really asking the children "open-ended" questions. . . . And she, Mertus, was not quite so late. . . . Ada Dixon still scowled: the improvements did not satisfy her. But a few months later, when she was responsible for the Employee Time Record, she applied the time policy most efficiently.

And the Mom and Tots day-care children who were old enough to enter school in the fall were encouraged to enroll in neighborhood Headstart programs during the summer.

Johnnie West, the VNA nurse Carol Howard, and a suburban obstetrician[3] who came during clinic once a week took care of the pregnant women.[4] Johnnie greeted them, served them juice and coffee, and talked with them "like a mother to an expectant mother," she said. She always had in mind her own experience with her baby Grace.

Glancing up at the red and blue and yellow and brown bulletin boards in the reception area, she used them as a guide for discussion. "HAVE A NORMAL BABY AND FEEL GOOD: BEFORE YOU ARE PREGNANT; DURING YOUR PREGNANCY; AFTER THE BABY". . . . "KEEP YOUR CHILDREN WELL". . . . After a few weeks, a guide was hardly necessary:

"It's good if you only get x rays in the ten days after your menstruation period, and the reason is the egg is not there then, so you can't be pregnant. If you are pregnant, and there is no way you can tell right at the beginning, the x rays might hurt the unborn child. . . .

"Foods like meat and milk and cheese and green leaf vege-
tables are good for you. . . . The darker the food is, the more
iron it has.

"Instead of a dessert that contains a lot of sugar, why not
a fruit, oranges, apricots, or something like this which is low
in calories and high in vitamins? . . .

"Some of the dangers of being overweight is your heart;
you have such a great load on your heart; and another dangerous thing, to me it's dangerous, you lose your identity because
all fat people look alike and this is not good for you. . . .

"If you suspect you are pregnant you should go to the
doctor so the doctor can check you for certain diseases and if
you have them he can give you treatments to clear them out
so they won't affect your baby and you can be healthy through
your pregnancy. Now for instance if you have ever been around
anyone with German measles you should go to the doctor
and he will give you an injection and the reason why: anyone
with German measles while they are pregnant it will affect
the baby . . . the same for venereal diseases, and diabetes;
and anemia, what you call low blood; and high blood pressure
too. . . .

"A lady should gain up to about twenty pounds and she
should gain it a pound a month for the first six months and
then the last three months she should try to gain about three
pounds a month which would be around twenty or maybe
under in the nine months of pregnancy. . . .

"Some of the signs to watch is swelling, for instance your
feet and your hands and around your eyes, if they get puffy;
and another sign is headaches and dizziness, this is a sign of
complications; and shortness of breath and cramps and bleeding. If you start bleeding before it is time to go to the hospital
you should tell your doctor about this. . . .

"Now you shouldn't complain too much about a low salt
diet; anything that the doctor or the nurse tell you to do you
should try because it's for your own good. And when the doctor puts you on a low salt diet this really means more than
stop using table salt, it means foods that contain salts or are
highly salty; and some of the foods would be potato chips,

crackers, salt pork, bacon, ham, cold cuts, these are the foods you should discontinue to use. . . .

"A lady should have a certain amount of exercise when she is pregnant and a certain amount of recreation; and it is important for the husband to pay her a little extra attention to help build up her ego, or he should take her out or just let her go out and maybe take walks, and that way she can enjoy plus have the exercise. . . .

"How long should a lady have intercourse while she is pregnant? Well now I would say maybe up to about eight months, if there are no complications, if she is healthy. She could ask her doctor and see what he says about it; and if the husband is willing to go along with her on this, because it's important, since we have a husband. . . .

"The lady who has never had a baby, how would they know when it's time? I think there are about three good signs. One is the show, if you start bleeding; another is if your water breaks; and another one is when you start having regular labor pains. . . .

"Even before your nine months you should already make arrangements on how you are going to get to the hospital and all this should be taken care of, plus you should have your clothes packed. . . . and if you have children at home you should make all the arrangements ahead of time and that way you can go to the hospital and just be comfortable, you don't have to be worrying or anything. . . .

"One way you can make labor much easier is abdominal breathing. We can practice this so you can get it down pat. One reason I always say is that it takes your mind off of labor, if nothing else. . . . I really think it helps—it helped me. . . .

"After you get home, one of the things you should watch out for are blood clots and excess bleeding. It should last maybe about three weeks, usually. You might also get cramps . . . or headaches or fever. . . .

"If a lady is not going to breast feed her baby and her breasts are full of milk, there are ways she can relieve the discomfort. One way will be to bandage and use ice packs. . . . She can get an old sheet and some pins and wrap herself tight, but not so tight as to stop circulation. . . . And if she doesn't have an ice bag she can always use plastic and wrap the ice up in plastic and apply this to her breasts . . . but she should never pop or massage her breasts because if you pop them or massage them this only increases the flow of milk the same way as if the baby was nursing from your breasts. . . .

"I really don't see why you should stay in the house for two weeks, because the baby needs a little air and so do you; but I believe if women have very set ideas about what she should do after delivery, if the woman or her family thinks she should stay in, I don't want to contradict them; I would leave it up to them to do what they think; anyway I don't think staying in the house is going to harm you, so it don't make too much difference. . . .

"And your six weeks' examination, this is important. You should go back. A lot of ladies don't, but I would say all of the ladies at the Mom and Tots have come back because we stress the point. This way the doctor can tell whether or not you are healthy and any complications. . . .

"Before the six week examination, a lot of ladies wonder if it is o.k. to have intercourse with their husbands, and can they get pregnant during that time. Yes, you can; and you should really wait until six weeks when the womb is healed. But in case you find it is impossible, you can buy different things at the drugstore; they have the rubber that the husband can use and if the husband would use a rubber and the lady would use a jelly, she would be almost as safe as if she was taking the pills or a coil or something. . . .

"A good time to space your children would be about fifteen months.[5] I think it takes at least a year before your body gets back together, and you have to start building your blood and everything up, so give yourself time to relax and take it easy. And if you would wait the fifteen months or two years or so, I guess the other child is just about able to take care of itself as far as feeding and toilet training and all that. . . ."

And when Johnnie had no answers for their questions, Carol Howard was always nearby.

In time, Johnnie was demonstrating how to bathe a baby and how to prepare a formula in the kitchen.

She asked the ladies to fill out a questionnaire[6] to guide the staff in planning group discussions during clinic. What did they already know? What did they want to know?

On the basis of their answers, Johnnie and the Mom and Tots staff, and the mothers and children joined in making a series of slides on Prenatal Care, Infant Care, and the Care of Young Children. Then the ladies in clinic could see what Johnnie was talking about, and so could the day-care mothers; they could see themselves. Johnnie also made use of a newly purchased animated slide series called How Babies Are Made. The prenatal patients found the slides helpful, even though they were designed for young children.

At the suggestion that the series be shown to the day-care children, Mertus was taken aback. She did not want "those sex slides" for the youngsters, animated or not. "I wouldn't know how to talk about them." Mrs. Jefferson and Ada were also affronted by the slides. Consequently, six months later, none of the children had seen any of them, not even the parts on plants and animals.

One day in late spring, Johnnie did not come to Clinic. Felecia, with uncoordinated enthusiasm, substituted.

The next week, Johnnie again did not come. She called. "I think I should quit. . . . I'm not dependable." She walked to the Center two days later. "I think you deserve an explanation. It's my husband. He doesn't want me to work. He wants me to stay with Grace, instead of my stepmother keeping her. . . . Seems like instead of getting closer together, we're getting farther apart. . . ."

Two weeks later Johnnie began bringing Grace with her to the Center. And Johnnie continued to work.

The clinic grew; twelve, fourteen, sixteen patients at the weekly sessions. A practical nurse began coming to help out from the VNA district office. A volunteer babysitter, an older woman usually, watched the patients' children during clinic. The younger women, those under twenty, came during the early part of the session, the older women came later. Some dropped in occasionally during the week, to check their weights, to ask questions, to chat.

The clinic grew. But the doctor said to keep it small. He wanted to be sure that no more than two hours of his time would be required. Mom and Tots was of no help to his private practice. . . . And he was going on summer vacation. Better have the patients return to the downtown hospital out-patient clinic.

But the patients were not sent downtown during his vacation; instead, a woman obstetrician came to take his place. Her manner sometimes frightened the patients. She told one woman she would die because of overweight, and another, a fifteen-year-old, she would hemorrhage because she refused to wear loose maternity clothes.

Carol Howard and Johnnie spent much time calming the ladies after the doctor left.

Sometimes women came in to say that the City obstetrical service (technically open to all who could not afford a private physician) would not accept them: they were too far along in their pregnancies—maybe six months and a half. This restriction by City health services was to "encourage" women to come for obstetrical care early in their pregnancies. The Center would call and make appointments for these women at the City-designated hospital; the Center said they were not so advanced— maybe five months and a half. Then, if deemed appropriate by the hospital clinic, the patients could return to the neighborhood clinic at Mom and Tots later.

Carol Howard visited the new babies at home within a week after delivery. And she kept in touch with mothers at two months, three months, and seven months after delivery.[7] She would ask how the baby was eating and whether he had had his shots. Did the mother want help getting him to the clinic? Was she back to normal? How was her child-spacing method working? And she was reminded to use the card Johnnie gave her for her wallet, with the baby's formula and the numbers to call for his check-up, and her birth control, and transportation service from Mom and Tots.[8]

The ladies began to ask whether they could get their birth control supplies at Mom and Tots? Mrs. Watkins was the first. "When am I gonna be able to get my pills at Mom and Tots? It's such a fuss to get downtown to the Planned Parenthood."

And Mertus thought she might take her pills more regularly if she could get them at Mom and Tots.

Since City health services did not help as they originally promised, the Planned Parenthood League agreed to furnish family planning services at Mom and Tots. Once a week they sent a gynecologist; a nurse, old Mrs. McGovern; and a volunteer from the suburbs, Mrs. Van Fleet.

Tommie Sanderson and his friends helped get the program started. They distributed the fliers: "Come to the Birth Control Clinic At Mom and Tots . . . complete physical examination . . . free pregnancy tests . . . call Mom and Tots for an appointment. . . ."[9]

Felecia was one of the first patients. After a reduced fee had been set,[10] Mrs. McGovern said, "But you didn't list your own job. The fee would have been more if you had, you know."

"Yes, I know," said Felecia, "that's why I didn't put down about my job."

Bewildered at her honesty, the nurse handed Felecia her six-month supply of pills.

Later, the Mom and Tots staff enjoyed the anecdote. Such stories were not uncommon.

One mother of six, who came in order to begin using a family planning method, asked whether her daughter Francine, fourteen, could get pills. Francine was "doing things" and she didn't want her getting "knocked up." Mrs. McGovern was unequivocal. "Planned Parenthood is not going to help girls be promiscuous!"[11]

Mom and Tots put Francine and her mother in contact with the City health services which were willing to help them.

By phone call and visit, the people around Kercheval and McClellan asked Mom and Tots for help.

"I got a sore tooth but they ain't no dentist around. . . ."

"My child needs his eyes checked. . . ."

"Can I get into a housing project?"

"I want to get pregnant, but I can't. . . ."

Lists of services were posted by the phones. And they

grew. Medical clinics, dental, eye, speech and hearing, family planning, gynecological, fertility; emergency food, clothing, shelter; V. D. treatment, TB x rays; poison control; day-care programs, preschools; public housing, Fair Housing Practices; legal and financial aid; job applications, job training. . . .

The staff faithfully followed the rule: if you don't know the answer, don't give one. Go find out.

One enjoyable way to find out was to role-play. Mrs. Watkins would be an old lady who needed food stamps. Ada Dixon would try to tell her how to apply for them. Mertus would caution, "Don't forget to ask her whether there's more people in her family."

Then Felecia would become a preschooler with a cut finger. Johnnie rendered first aid and then called his mother. "Lord have mercy," Ada laughed, "Felecia, you raise more fuss than Little Darrell and Danny put together."

Someone else would become a mother whose sixteen-year-old was pregnant.

And so they learned the *official* way to use the "system."

There were other sessions to talk over situations such as: You see a young child pounding another youngster with a brick. While holding the child, what should you say to him?

(1) "I know you are angry, but we don't want anyone to be hurt."

(2) "I'm surprised at you! Good little boys don't hit other little boys."

(3) "While you are in day care, you will have to behave yourself."

(4) "Why are you hitting that nice little boy?"

The father of a boy two and a half years old says to you, "Please don't give Billy any dolls to play with, even if he asks for them. I don't want him to be a sissy." What should you answer?

(1) "Children of Billy's age do not yet know the difference between male and female behavior."

(2) "Billy would not play with dolls if you spent more time with him."

(3) "I agree with you that Billy should play with toys that are made especially for boys."

A three-year-old boy draws a picture and says to you, "It kitty." Which response should you give?

(1) "A kitty has more than two legs."

(2) "Why yes, you have made a picture of a kitty. Does the kitty have a name?"

(3) "Wonderful! It's the most beautiful cat I ever saw!"

(4) "I'll draw a cat for you. Then you can copy it."[12]

More important than the answers were the reasons behind the answers, and the discussions and thoughts which flowed from them, on discipline, on sexuality, on the meaning of growth.

There were other discussions, spontaneous ones, like the time Tommie Sanderson sneaked into day care, and Mertus yelled at him and pushed him out. He pounded on the front window until they thought it would break.

Why was Tommie so angry?

"He's just mean and ugly," said Ada.

"But he's not always that way," Johnnie reminded them. "Like for instance, yesterday. He made some kind of ice cream for the other children by freezing some milk and sugar in the ice trays."

It was true that Tommie had behavior problems. But how would they feel if there were nine other children in their family and no one had much time for them? And people were always pushing them away?

"I might think there's something wrong with me maybe. And I don't think I'd like those people either," thought Felecia.

Now Mom and Tots had thrown him out, too.

"Well, I guess I can see why he is so angry," said Mrs. Watkins. "But he sure can't be in day care."

That was true. But perhaps they could explain *why* to him. And if they understand why he gets angry, perhaps they in turn won't have to get angry themselves.

Ada had a wry look. And Mertus nodded affirmatively without expression on her face.

From the beginning, the children came. They wanted to play after school; six-eight-ten-twelve-year-olds. Who could watch out for them?

Almost as early, the teenagers came. Someone at ACME had said Mom and Tots was hiring babysitters.

The teens began to meet once a week to talk about what babies are like, and children, and people. They set Rules for Baby Sitters:

(1) NEVER leave children alone.

(2) One child only in each crib.

(3) Always keep crib rails up.

(4) Change crib sheet after each baby.

(5) DIAPERING:
Wash skin with Dial soap.
Put used diapers in a plastic bag to go home.
Use A & D ointment and disposable diapers.
Change wet clothes.

(6) FEEDING:
Refrigerate milk.
Use bottle-warmer.
Throw out unused portion of milk.
Small children should not have peanuts or popcorn.

(7) Children are not allowed in the kitchen.

(8) Children may play in the window if supervised.

(9) REMEMBER: Children Are Important:
　　　　　　　　Talk to them
　　　　　　　　Listen to them
　　　　　　　　Play with them
　　　　　　　　Love them
　　　　　　　　They want the same things you want.

The teens sat from 3:30 to 5 for seventy-five cents in the day-care area. That was free-play for the school-aged children, the six- to twelve-year-olds.

At their meetings, other questions came up among the eight or ten or twelve of them. They saw Hank, slow in mind and body. What was wrong with him? A discussion followed about birth defects, and basic health before pregnancy, and early treatment of disease.

And there were other questions:

How old do you think a girl should be before she starts having babies?

How old do you think a girl should be when she gets married?

I want to know about pregnancy and how it will feel.

What do you think about boys using protection? (condom)

Why do most boys get hard by kissing?

WHy do most boys like to have relationship most of the time when they are with their girl friends?

Some questions were put to them in hours of discussion over cookies and milk:

How many ways are there for people to be intimate with each other?

Why do people like to be intimate?

Why might some people not like to be intimate?

How many people have you been close to?

Why do people engage in sexual intimacy? How many reasons for it are there besides wanting to have babies?

What responsibilities do people have when they are intimate? How do you want to be treated when you are close to someone?

What added responsibilities are there when people are intimate sexually?

How can you prepare yourself to fulfill these responsibilities? . . .

Some discussions were on food, what they ate, how to prepare it.

A day's fare might be:

breakfast	rice with bacon
	grape drink
dinner	sloppy joe's
	coke
in between	potato chips
	coke

Or

breakfast	eggs
	sausages
	grits
	juice
dinner	baked chicken
	cabbage
	corn bread
	milk
in between	ice cream
	cookies

At other times it was cigarette-smoking, menstruation, venereal disease.

As the babysitters became the Babysitters Club and then the Teen Club,[13] the meetings were enriched by visits from a fashion expert, a Negro artist, meal parties; in addition, there were visits to Motown, live theaters, and public buildings. They made sure "health" would not be confined to a narrow definition.

One phone call to Mrs. Jefferson and she had a dozen pre-teen girls in a club at Mom and Tots within a week. They elected officers and learned to knit and crochet quietly. But they liked cooking, too, and some even whispered about ministration (menstruation).

She just knew their mothers wouldn't approve if she talked about *that*.

After about six months, Mrs. Jefferson was calling some twenty mothers of her pre-teens. "Why they actually sounded relieved. They said they didn't know how they would talk to their girls about it."

She borrowed a film, got some booklets, wrote a test on "Hygiene":

> Spell the name of the subject you have been studying about. . . .
>
> Where did the word originate? . . .
>
> Meaning what? . . .
>
> Will this occur each month around the same day? . . .
>
> Can you perform your usual duties at this time? . . .
>
> Would you wear a white dress at this time? . . .
>
> Would you dispose of pads in the toilet? . . .
>
> Have you started your period yet? . . .
>
> Would you like to know more about your body, and how it will grow in the next few years? If so, you may

attend our next lectures on anatomy and physiology of the female reproductive organs.[14]

Soon cooking lessons and crafts were added to Mrs. Jefferson's curriculum.

But some young girls didn't like to sit and knit. They mobilized around a mop and pail in a basement "Clean-up Party" with Carol Howard's help. So began a second Girls Club with one of the older teenagers as sponsor. Games and dancing and sports were on their agenda.

And some girls went to both Clubs each week.

Everyone knew the young boys needed a man. Two or three or four dozen little boys came to the Center after school, and more did so in the summer.

Ada Dixon had a neighbor, a young man of twenty, the oldest of fifteen children. He would soon be part of the regular summer lay off at the Chrysler plant.

Within two days, Regi Conrad was on the job as Boys' Club sponsor, ten hours a week at Mom and Tots. Tall and lean, he was as gentle as he could be rough, as much a boy as a man.

He set up a schedule:

Monday—Baseball

Tuesday—Swimming

Wednesday—Indoors

Thursday—Exercises

Friday—Free play

with ice cream or milk or juice and molasses cookies afterward.

"Indoors" sometimes meant talking about why the boys didn't like school, or how fires start, or why they shouldn't smoke. The boys answered:

Cigarette-smoking brings on lung cancer and heart diseases. . . . You can die from it. . . .

Tar and nicotine are poisons in cigarettes. . . .

People who have habits like smoking are trying to kill themself. . . .

Dope will kill you too. . . .

Or it meant being weighed and measured, and having teeth, eyes, and ears looked at. Sometimes it meant parties and dancing.

They made up their Rules of the Boys' Club:

1. Please come in hang up coats and sit down.

2. *NO* piano playing (or pay a five-cent fine).

3. Keep hands to yourselves.

4. Please do not talk out of turn.

5. When an officer of the club or the counselor says to stop (PLEASE STOP).

6. Don't run around in the club, you may injure yourself.

7. *NO* fighting, yelling, or using profanity.

8. Do *NOT* go in the kitchen.

9. Try to come as *NEAT* as possible.

10. Do not leave the club without permission (except in case of emergency).

11. *NO* playing in the windows.

12. *NO* gum chewing while playing.

13. Please try not to call anyone out of their name. (This means to address people by proper names, not "Hey you." N.M.)

It was an effort at reasonable authority, self-discipline based on mutual respect. Regi thought about some of these things himself. Sure he knew the boys needed to learn to take care of themselves. But he got mad sometimes; no one ever was patient with *him*.

Sometimes the Mom and Tots staff would be mother to whole families, to people the official agencies labeled "unresponsive to teaching," "unresponsive to children's needs," "very slow to follow instructions," "uncooperative." Mrs. Bailey and her children were one of those families. On official welfare records her problems were listed as

1. Needed postnatal exam and family planning for Mrs. Bailey.
2. Needed postnatal exam and family planning for daughter Charlene.
3. Immunizations for Yolanda, Brian, and Gerald.
4. Medical examination and immunizations for Tracey (granddaughter).
5. Medical examination and treatment for Mrs. Bailey.

At the Center Mertus enrolled preschooler Yody Bailey in day care. Her mother smiled broadly and went back to the kitchen table, chatting with Mrs. Watkins. "You know, I been looking all over for a place to keep her. . . . These legs of mine, they sure do pain me sometimes". . . . Mrs. Watkins listened closely.

Mrs. Watkins knew that Mrs. Bailey was not "uncooperative" or "unresponsive to her children's needs." It was just that she could not get to all the clinics that the health people wanted her to go to. Her energies were directed first at getting food and clothes for her children and grandchildren. Considering her own ill-health, there was little energy left to locate the proper clinics or to coordinate the sheer mechanical arrangements: finding someone to sit with the younger children most of the day, getting transportation to the clinics, remembering to bring food along for the youngsters she would have to take with her, and squeezing all this between the hours after some of the children left for school in the morning and prior to the supper hour for her son who left for work in the afternoon. To contemplate attempting all this five times, for each of the five prescribed clinic visits, was just too much for Mrs. Bailey.

Mrs. Watkins understood this. She casually called upstairs and asked Johnnie West, Ada Dixon, and the nurse Carol Howard to join them at coffee.

Soon, they were on the phones, making appointments and arranging transportation, with assenting nods from Mrs. Bailey. Medical examinations were set for the children at a no-charge pediatric clinic. Mrs. Bailey was to have her medical examination at a no-charge adult clinic. On the clinic dates, Ada had a driver pick up the Baileys to transport them to the doctor while the remaining youngsters were watched at the Center.

Two weeks later, the family planning procedure was easily arranged through the services available at Mom and Tots.

Within a month all Mrs. Bailey's problems, as officially listed, were solved.

Sometimes Mom and Tots could change the feelings of those who were afraid of medical people.

One of the teenage boys saw a two-year-old fall in the alley and cut her leg. He carried her upstairs to Mom and Tots. She began to cry and was cared for on Carol Howard's lap. Her six-year-old sister took her home. A few minutes later they returned with four other children and stuck their heads in the door.

Why had they come back?

"Oh, just to see." They all grinned.

Three months after Open House, and the summer got hotter. More flies. More roaches. More calls to Rilka Vasiloff; more of her promises—for a screen door, a fumigator. Little satisfaction.

More people. More children. More complexity.

Mary Louise Moore, a practical nurse, came to help. She would relieve Carol Howard eight hours a week. Carol Howard was feeling the call to greater responsibility through the more established channels of her profession.

Mary Louise Moore worked in the district office of the VNA; the routine work didn't demand much of—or develop —her creative energies. She had dark brown skin and big black eyes that could glow with warmth or anger, or be vacant of feeling. At will, she could turn out the world or let it in to see her deep aesthetic sensibilities. She was somewhat of a paradox, with a large voluptuous bosom and a shy gracious manner. She agreed to "try" at Mom and Tots with the uncertainty and courage of an almost existential leap.

Mary Louise, now in her early thirties, had grown up in the neighborhood in a church-going family; one nephew was aspiring to be a concertmaster; a sister was the first Negro to enter one of the wealthier suburbs. Mary Louise had a year of college, but had not wanted to continue there.

She moved slowly into the programs, helping in the prenatal clinic, leading monthly sessions with the children's groups, helping to guide Regi, arranging transportation for mothers, trying to help Mertus get organized.

One day, looking astounded, she referred to the private conversations of the staff: "Everyone is either '*black*' or '*white*'. . . . 'White people don't know what our children need. . . .' It's always 'we' and 'they. . . .' " She had even overheard someone ask, "What side is Mary Louise on?"

Mary Louise said she wasn't used to conversation like that. She always got along with white people.

Was this naiveté? Or denial? Or the well-known Negro art of indirection?[15]

The summer got warmer and more alive. One evening Felecia and the old Irish cook, who came on invitation, headed a Food Demonstration with the rest of the staff for neighborhood women:

Find out
>—how to stretch your food budget
>—short cuts to fixing meals
>—how to fix children's foods

Mrs. Watkins described how she made cornbread. A nutritionist who came from the VNA passed out some liver recipes: liver loaf, liver patties, liver stew, liver chop suey, liver casserole, liver with brown gravy, with sauce, with onions, Spanish liver, chicken livers. And a few cookie recipes—oatmeal, peanut, molasses, whole wheat. The dozen mothers who came said they enjoyed the coffee and conversation.

Another evening the day-care mothers and staff had a Moms, Tots, and Pops Nite:

> a window showcase of entertainment
> for the whole family:
> dances,
> songs,
> singalongs,
> poetry,
> puppets,
> and refreshments.

Mertus was mistress of ceremonies. The storefront was filled. Music overflowed. Rev. Clay Shaw rushed over from Allan Temple across the street, "Ladies, *please*, we're trying to have a conference." So the amplifier was taken inside.

The Mothers Clubs of the two neighboring preschools, one Catholic-sponsored, the other under public-school auspices, visited Mom and Tots. They wanted to know about first aid, and weight control, and birth control. Mostly birth control. "Why didn't they tell us this *before* we were pregnant?" Several came to the Mom and Tots birth control clinic. One came to the prenatal clinic.

The summer was warmer and more fervid.

Alfred, from A C M E, walked briskly over to the Center with two others. "The people in the community want to know how you get into this place." He heard. And they left.

The leader from the Freedom Now Party came over. Removing his hat, he looked around, and began to talk about birth control. The pills were not safe. The government was giving experimental pills to poor people. The white power structure was using birth control to control Black people.

In response, he was asked how Mom and Tots could force people to do what they didn't want to do.

He didn't answer that. He talked on for an hour.

Looking around again he said, "It's a nice place you got here." He put on his hat and left.

An ACME boy was shot by two white men in a car, it was said. Luke came over to the Center to ask whether anyone had seen anything. No one had.

The corner bank was robbed one afternoon. The police came over to the Center to ask whether anyone had seen anything. No one had.

Mrs. Pete Collins Jackson came to Mom and Tots with a son, an ACME member, to speak for her contractor-husband whose whereabouts were unknown. Where was the money for the "extra charges" her husband asked for? She was cold fury.

The matter was in the hands of lawyers. The subcontractors took it to them.

She stalked out with loud curses.

Two hours later, Luke came over with another Jackson son. What was this all about? Had Mr. Jackson been screwed?

Luke heard the details and he was given the phone numbers of the VNA lawyers.

He never mentioned the matter again.

The summer was warmer and more complex.

The problem of maintaining some degree of communication with ACME and the views it held was discussed with a leader of the Friends of the Northern Student Movement. He suggested, as a part-time worker, a young woman who had worked for the Student Nonviolent Coordinating Committee in Selma and had recently returned to Detroit. She was finishing college and she needed a place. He brought her to talk.

Laine Thomas was stylishly thin, dressed in browns over her black skin. She wore sunglasses indoors when talking to white people whom she didn't trust, which meant most white people. She spoke with a mildly East Coast accent, having gone to school there. She came quickly to the point. The Mom and Tots Center needed a youth worker. She could do that.

She needed a position from which to help coordinate "The

Movement" between the East and West sides of the City. She knew Luke Pride. She would work with him.

So Laine took the Teen Club and the "active" preteens. A Black bookstore became their supply source. The younger ones began using "Color Me Brown" books, and the teenagers had their first taste of Black underground theater.

They responded immediately to Laine's approach:

> I think that a person's image of himself is probably the most important thing that a person carries with him through life. . . . As soon as you start talking about poor people, especially poor black people, you don't realize how important this kind of concept is until you realize the effect that it has on somebody who looks in the mirror and sees that he doesn't have on a white hat or does not have white skin. . . . I would like to provide a place where this negative image is not reinforced . . . not necessarily changed. . . . I think this is a very bad concept to grow up with. . . . The way that I think I am doing that or trying to do that is . . . providing an atmosphere where the girls can do things themselves. The basis is that they can do beautiful things and are not imposed with a fantastic amount of discipline. . . .[16]

The girls were responding to Laine.

But what about the staff? What about Mary Louise? Would they be able to work with Laine?

Because the Center would be losing Carol Howard, its part-time visiting nurse, it sent letters to SNCC, the Congress on Racial Equality, NSM, the Urban League, the Southern Christian Leadership Conference, and the NAACP in search of another.

The prospective nurses who visited the Center expressed their views in their first comments:

> Why, when everyone else is working for integration, do you want to hire a *Negro* nurse? . . .

> I work midnights now. Would there be evening work or weekends? . . .

I belong to CORE, SNCC, and NAACP, but I'm not very militant. . . . I'm thirty-six now, and I'm more realistic than I used to be. . . . I know what you can do and what you can't do. . . . I would've been interested in this ten years ago. . . .

The search would continue for another year.

Early in the fall the staff gathered around the big kitchen table behind the counter for the weekly meeting. Mertus was having some abdominal pains; what could she do? "Betcha didn't take your birth control like you should've," teased Felecia.

Mrs. Watkins was faithfully taking her iron pills.

Ada reported that Mrs. Vasiloff had not yet turned on the heat.

Hank was coming home this week from the rehabilitation center. His legs had been treated with wedging casts even though the doctor had said that "because of his poor IQ and poor cultural background, he's not worth the money to treat him." Now the VNA would help him at home until he could learn to walk again. Carol Howard would supervise that personally.

Felecia presented a picture she had drawn for a new Mom and Tots flier—a mother and children in cartoon with the features of a Caucasian ideal-type.

"Well, what's wrong with it?" she asked, looking around.

"Now you know we don't look like that—not that I think it matters," said Mertus.

"Oh. . . . I wondered about that. . . . You want me to do it over, huh? . . . Well, O.K."

Her next attempt was the one used on the stencil.

Mom and Tots had received an offer from the Junior League, a service society of well-to-do women. They would be willing to sing Christmas carols and bring Santa to the children at Mom and Tots at Christmastime.

Ada Dixon thought that was very nice of them. Mrs. Watkins thought the children might enjoy music.

Mertus was reluctant. "We have our own talent. . . . Our churches have their own choirs. . . . What do the 'Great White Mothers' have that we don't?"

Laine thought that even considering the idea was distasteful.

The Junior League was thanked and was refused.

Mom and Tots would plan its own Christmas party with a Black Santa.

Ada looked up from the newspaper which often accompanied her to staff meeting. In exasperation she said, "You all do what you want." She hunched down again.

The
staff
and

I worked side by side, literally, as the facets of the Center unfolded; we worked slowly, closely, constantly. At first I joined them in talking to the women and, sometimes, men who came to enroll children in day care, or to enter the clinics, or for an increasing number of other reasons. And then we would talk about what we had done. I helped them see where they were not listening before they answered; and they helped me understand where I was not hearing, as at the time they thought I had embarrassed a husband by discussing birth control with his wife. They needed to know what I could see as an observer; I needed to understand what they knew by intuition. Both kinds of awareness shaped the direction, the types and tone of the Center's programs. Gradually, they took on most of the direct contact with neighborhood people, bringing to me what they did not feel comfortable doing on their own; my desk was set purposely out of the way in one area of the second floor. Regularly and together we would look at the day's events.

Mertus was the most articulate or, more accurately, the most facile with words; for words did not seem to flow out of her as an expression of herself. After many encounters with her I began to understand how she *used* words to manipulate situations and people: for a long while I was led to believe that her understanding of social and psychological processes was equal to her ability to use terms which the others did not use, such as "identity," "motivation," "aggression." I do not make this observation as a judgment, for words are commonly used in this way, potentially separating us from ourselves and each other; and, we would probably say, better for a person to try to manipulate his environment with words than with force. However, for Mertus as a human being, this veneer of words was detrimental. She did not know her self. Through her facility with words, her self became the one that was most politically advantageous to a situation, sometimes Negro and sometimes "white," apparently permissive or punitively restrictive, sexually inviting or Victorian in attitude, cajoling of authority or extremely hostile to it. She could not focus herself and was afraid to look and try.

Her uncertainty about what she really was or wanted to be, her ambivalence and insecurity, was reflected both in her desire for external controls for herself, such as "docking," and in her desire to control others: she wanted the children and the staff women to obey her without question. The conception of authority implicit in her behavior was authoritarian and quantitative. Authority was almost a quantity bestowed on one person to which other people then acceded, rather than the result of a reciprocal relationship aimed at achieving mutually valued goals.

Thus, discipline for herself could not come from within, because she could not be certain what was there. New circumstances, without rigid rules, were especially frightening. She preferred to have the rules set up first rather than act in an unstructured situation and develop the necessary rules on the basis of what appeared to be needed: it was the difference between the development of arbitrary and of rationally based authority as well as external and internal control.

Her facility with language allowed her to absorb the terminology in her environment so that she could *talk* for example, about self-discipline and maintaining a free environment for the children; but she could not consistently *act* on this basis because she could not psychologically tolerate it.

What in her own behavior appeared to be permissiveness was really a lack of self-discipline, a wildness of sorts, a kind of malignant self-expression, rather than the real permissiveness which flows from inner freedom and security, a certainty of one's self. She could not discipline her imagination sufficiently, most of the time, to make it reality.

Because Mertus liked to use words and could talk very well, we had long conversations as the months went by. She seemed to understand in discussion the meaning of authority, and eventually she could admit to me some of her personal ambivalences, but in front of the other women she refused to admit to any uncertainties or mistakes, refused to "be herself," saying this would undermine her authority. In fact a look of fear came into her eye—the one seeing eye—at the thought of exposing herself to the others; she could not allow others to see what she herself feared to look at.

It was important for me to try to help Mertus begin to look at herself and at her understanding of authority, for she was to supervise other women, and her personality would pervade the day-care program. Even beyond that, the basic question of the meaning of authority and discipline was implicit in so much of what happened within and around the Center. The essence of the question was always, shall we move toward a rationally based authority, growing out of internal controls, self-discipline, inner freedom, or toward an arbitrary authority based on external controls, the "do-it-because-I-say-so" approach? And if we seek the former for ourselves, how shall we act to make the same thing possible for those we are working with?

Mertus' behavior did not change with the passage of time, as did that of Felecia and Mrs. Watkins and the others. Mertus could not see that they would remain divided from her if she did not give more of her self to them and accept from them what they offered. I realized how unsuited she was psychologically for her job. She ended her own role at the Center, the only person to leave, a year later (see Part 5).

But on a less analytic, perhaps less philosophical and more practical level, Mertus had many characteristics which were important to the development of the Center, in addition to what I learned through relating to her. Like many innovative-types, she was willing to dream, to try new things in spite of her fears, to confront and test authority, as she often did with me, demanding for instance a half hour coffee break, complaining about equipment, calling me anytime from 6 A.M. to 1 A.M.; and she would use her language facility in describing to me the feelings and attitudes of her friends. Her perceptions and interpretations were very helpful, even though they were reshaped at times to suit her own interests. Although I could never be sure of her purposes, at least her position was consistently that of a person intent on manipulating "the system," which, inevitably, I represented, especially in the beginning months. Her position was a legitimate one for the ghetto dweller, one, therefore, I wanted to be aware of.

Her confrontations with me about pictures from *McCall's* or *Ebony*, about coffee breaks, or about inadequate supplies, in the first days of the Center before I knew any of them as individual personalities, helped me see myself more clearly in relation to the staff. Through her complaints about supplies, for instance, it became clear to me that if the staff could manage their own portions of the budget, having the same financial constraints that I had to deal with, they could then heap upon themselves whatever praise or blame resulted from the spending of the funds: They could stretch the funds and feel both the satisfactions and frustrations of that kind of control.

Moreover, Mertus' refusal to think through what would be done at the first official day-care session made me realize that I would need to let go, to allow certain things to happen which were against my better judgment. In this case the anxiety Mertus felt at that first session was a far stronger impetus to future planning on her part than any admonition I could have given.

In learning, and relearning, to view an incident from more than one perspective, I recognized that there is no single "answer," no "best" way that I from one vantage point could dictate, no matter what my educational or professional credentials.

On the other hand, I realized there were some situations— such as using black faces from *Ebony* instead of white faces from *McCalls* on the bulletin boards—where I would uphold my own value commitments regardless of the staff's opinions. In this instance, as was my practice, I first tried to discuss the problem with

Mertus as the others watched. I used an indirect approach; attempting to have her question her assumption that "it's up to the Negro to adjust to the white world." My words at that point were futile. And I finally told her, in unmasked exasperation and anger, to use the pictures from *Ebony*. Then I left.

It was at about this time I began to realize that although I am white, I am not all wrong. Although my race is responsible for degrading other races, I do not bear the guilt alone or as an individual; I can accept my responsibility for working toward human wholeness in society out of a sense of personal conviction and worth rather than self-recrimination and guilt. On this basis I can stand in agreement or disagreement with any man, black or white, and in quietude or anger. I began to realize that as in any other relationships, but especially between black and white, infinite patience is no more conducive to wholeness than perpetual rage, expressed or hidden. Dishonest patience or tolerance is as belittling as open disdain.

These awarenesses became clear to me not many days after the Center opened in April. Prior to that time my diary reflected a gradual change in my responses, which I was not aware of at the time. At first the days were "fascinating. . . . how beautifully, incredibly complex. . . . I did good battle with Pete Jackson and crew today . . . was badgered by ACME today. . . . another adventure . . . it would take a book to go through the day." Then, "many brick walls for me to ram and people waiting to pick up the pieces, in the agencies and at the Center. . . . The difficulties in the project become fearsome when I get tired and beat out. . . . I am feeling alone and easily lose my perspective; so many difficulties to cope with. . . . Today I was on the verge of tears from 2 o'clock on. . . . this is my first awareness of what they call 'culture shock'. . . ."

For many weeks I had seen my professional colleagues only occasionally. For reasons I have described, they regarded me as wanting "to do things the hard way." And, I had discarded my blue uniform, which was, in a profession which is recognized by, and recognizes itself by, its uniforms, another barrier to my communication with them.

Thus, cut off and having cut myself off from what had been

familiar, and being in effect a stranger, an outsider, at the Center, "culture shock" was probably as inevitable as it was unexpected to me.

However, finally having some understanding of what was happening inside me, my feelings began to change almost immediately. I began expressing myself more directly to the staff, my anger and frustrations, as well as my pleasure in them, sometimes in mild four letter words, sometimes through joking. And they began to return similar feelings in the same ways. Gradually, first names were used; this was common practice after about fifteen to eighteen months, although I continued to use "Mrs." with the older women.

Johnnie West's limitations seemed to be more outside her than within her, in the constraints imposed by her husband and their economic circumstances, a state of affairs common to many ghetto women. As I became aware of her increasing problems at home, all I could do was let her know that the Center wanted and needed her and that we would try to arrange whatever she thought would help her most. She suggested bringing her baby Grace with her and so she did. Other people on the staff from time to time also helped mold the Center to their family circumstances. Again, this had importance beyond solving an immediate problem; it meant the Center could respond to living problems common to many other ghetto families.

Johnnie seemed to remember everything she heard, everything I had ever said to her in the days when I visited her house before Grace was born. She not only remembered, but related new things to old, asked questions, quietly observed, integrated her observations and expressed them again in new forms, relevant to new circumstances. Johnnie was the model in my mind of a translator of culture. She took knowledge, language, and methods from my culture of the health professional, educated, language-oriented, white, and reinterpreted these in the language and other forms of communication that made sense to members of her culture: lay, nonprofessional, less educated, less language-oriented, black. Together we tried to select the kinds of information which could have an impact on the lives of women who came as patients to the clinics. Together, with the rest of the staff and some of the patients, we worked out audio-visual means for communicating ideas. The very means of developing the slides and films was a ground for communication, for teaching and learning.

The more people could be a part of the process, the more color, feeling, and dramatics could be brought in, the better was the result, in communication, clarity, and pleasure. In other words, the Center used a less language-oriented mode for communication.

The Center itself had been created to listen and respond to the people of the neighborhood. Each clinic session and each basic program set up on a group basis attempted to meet the needs of those who formed it. In time, at the suggestions and urging of mothers and children, new facets of the Center unfolded. Except for our readiness, much of what happened had not been planned originally: the evening and weekend events, the clubs, most of what followed the next year, even the birth-control clinic would have been delayed without their impetus. It would have seemed an absurdity, just a few months before, for a Visiting Nurse Association to propose to sponsor what was now becoming the essence of the Center, a focus on wholeness increasingly removed from the traditional conception of "health."

What the Mom and Tots staff, for example, could do for Mrs. Bailey in a few days, official health structures had not been able to do after years of effort. The staff understood Mrs. Bailey's priorities, the problems which necessarily absorbed most of her energies, and the Center was fashioned to help her deal with them. If official health people could understand Mrs. Bailey's worries about food and clothing and uncertain income, they had not set up their agencies to help her realistically deal with them, so she remained to them "uncooperative," unable to use the existing health services.

As the people at the Center tried out their ideas, new ideas came to them. New arrangements yielded new perspectives, and new ways of seeing brought more ideas and more changes. Almost invariably, the first phases of any new program were paid for through donated time, talent, and money, since budgeted funds for these did not exist. But the greatest obstacle to developing new ideas was the lack of belief that one's own tentative and uncertain suggestions were sufficiently worthy to be tried out. Once this inertia of disbelief began to be overcome through a few experiences, once people saw that it was very acceptable to talk, to dream, to venture, new ideas began to mushroom. The atmosphere pulled newness from all of us.

Other health professionals were present at the Center for the short periods of time when their direct services were needed. Especially during the first year, except for Carol Howard, they did not come willingly. There are many complex reasons for this which may someday be the story of another book.

Contacts between the Center and ACME continued to be sporadic. The episode with Luke, following my encounter with Mrs. Pete Collins Jackson over contracting funds, meant to me that at least ACME knew we were trying to play the game straight. But it was obvious that I would personally be in an increasingly poor position to be conversant with ACME.

Although the Center's programs seemed to be developing very satisfactorily in the eyes of most neighborhood people, I thought the Center should have the benefit of the continuing perspective of militants, those who are conscious of having no interest in the status quo. Granted, their perspective was no more "objective" than anyone else's, but it was another way of seeing what was happening and thus essential to the Center.

At that time, Mary Louise was not the person to provide a line of sight with ACME. I had met her a few years earlier at the VNA district office and had talked with her occasionally. She was the kind of person you learn to know by inference. Thus, what I knew of her I felt sure of; but I did not know how much I did not know. I felt certain that because she had made the decision to come to the Center, this was a serious matter for her, that she believed in it as something that ought to be tried. That was her major qualification, as it was for everyone else. From that point on, she just needed time and a place to set free what was behind her eyes.

However, her experiences with militant black people, if

any, had been fewer than mine. And her contact in recent years with low-income black people was less than mine. In her first months at the Center she never used the words "black" or even "Negro" in talking to me. She would use "them," referring to the staff, or "us," meaning Negro people, or even vaguer references. Slowly I sought to make her use more explicit terms. I could not know then whether she was dealing with her personal discomfort and uncertainty about blackness, or whether she was intentionally withholding from me. In any case, she was not ready to be a link to ACME.

But Laine was. Although she was no more than about ten or fifteen years younger than Mary Louise, she was part of a different generation. Her dilemmas and ambivalences were of a different order. She had no doubts about how she felt toward what I represented. Her needs and purposes coincided for a time with those of the Center, and so she came. I think both our purposes were well served, although considering her ideological stance, Laine would be the first to tell me not to speak for her.

Laine also served an unanticipated purpose, beyond providing a line of communication with ACME, beyond criticizing the Center from a black militant point of view, beyond providing a model for the young girls of how the new black woman ought to think and act and look. In time she helped reveal to Mary Louise beauty in blackness, separating it from the poverty and ignorance with which it was bound in Mary Louise's thoughts and feelings. She helped make militancy a fact of life with which in time Mary Louise could communicate openly and directly.

Although I did not doubt the necessity of having someone like Laine at the Center, I worried whether she might have too divisive an effect. As always, the best safety valve would be group discussion. I hoped the staff would talk about their feelings together—their fear of black militancy, their discomfort in Laine's presence. And I hoped they would communicate their uncertainties, their suggestions, their reactions, to me. I knew they were learning that they could not change the shape of things by avoiding the power structure. Confronting authority figures together and with definitiveness was the only way they would gain a significant share of the power to shape their world.

The various staff members were not equally ready to confront the white world as black people; this was clearly revealed in the incident over Felecia's stencil and in their disagreement over accepting a Christmas party given by the Junior League. The League had asked my permission to give the party. In the eyes of the Center, of course, neither "yes" nor "no" could have been the "right" answer if *I* had given it. And to the ears of the Junior League, "no" was probably an affront. Thus, almost no one was happy about the decision when it was made.

Interestingly, I enjoyed the whole episode. I was beginning to appreciate the irony of varying perspectives, and was not quite so uncomfortable at being caught in the middle. Most of all, their decision to refuse the Junior League party, though not unanimous, was to me a hopeful sign. This had been the first open discussion among the whole staff in eight months about "black" and "white." It took place in front of me. And no one seemed especially uncomfortable.

The Center's Christmas party at the end of the first year was regarded as an overwhelming success. There was a part to play for everyone: mothers, fathers, children, all the clubs, even Laine and her girls, and Ada was in her red dress. The outcome belonged to them.

That first year revealed unquestioned potential for wholeness, but it also made clear grave threats to unfolding.

IV
Barriers

The Center sometimes could mother people, it sometimes could allay suspicions and fears, but sometimes it had a painful time taking care of itself.

Its energies, the thrust toward unfolding, could be dissipated by its own voices of mistrust, intolerance, anger.

From Ada Dixon:

Felecia is using the food budget to buy her own groceries.

Felecia is lazy.

Mertus is messy; she doesn't keep schedules straight.

The mothers don't like Mertus.

Mrs. Jefferson will give toys to the Center, but not to Mertus

The children are stealing us blind.

From Mertus:

Ada scares the children.

Ada is undermining her relationship with the mothers.

Felecia relies on her mother too much.

From Felecia:

Mertus is too critical.

Mertus doesn't help clean up.

Mertus is husband-stealing.

Mrs. Watkins takes everything too personal.

From Mrs. Watkins:

"I knew she wasn't our kind"—when she saw Laine talking to Luke at ACME (now AAYM, the Afro-American Youth Movement).

From Regi:

Felecia never pays her bets.

From Mary Louise:

Silence.

From Laine:

The pocket Community Directory the Center was preparing for the neighborhood was incomplete; you had to explain to people *how* to break through the system; it would take a year to write it properly; she didn't have the time.

Tommie Sanderson had too much freedom; he was just taking advantage of whitey; she didn't have time to show the sitters how they should discipline.

Mrs. Bailey needed more than medical help; she needed help to fight Welfare for additional money to support her many children.

Finally, Mertus called for an Evaluation Conference. What activities in the programs had been successful? What problems had they had with mothers and children? Which approaches were easiest for them? Which were hardest? It sounded like a complete agenda.

"But what we need," Felecia finally put it into words, "is a better spirit of cooperation". . . . She began by talking about herself. The others joined in.

Then they said Mertus needed to be a stronger leader.

They needed to share responsibility more.

Perhaps Ada would be happier if her work were moved upstairs.

The atmosphere was freer. After the meeting, Mrs. Watkins spoke to Laine, "Would you all mind getting me one of them ice cream cones?"

Eventually, Laine got legal aid for Mrs. Bailey and helped her through a court fight with Welfare.

Ada Dixon took Regi aside and helped him apologize to Felecia for their misunderstanding on the bet.

Ada's typewriter was moved into the second-floor kitchen. She continued, as she had been for years, on tranquilizers, but in diminishing doses and with fewer migraines.

And the children continued to help themselves to cookies and raisins and milk first, and ask permission afterward.

Mary Louise had her first conversation with Luke Pride. One afternoon, while she was arranging her "Neighborhood Notes" bulletin board in the window, he walked across the street. One of his A A Y M women needed a place to leave her child, and a temporary shelter; her house had burned. Mary Louise knew what to do.

Thereafter, she and Luke had conversations about policing the police, and about how Luke might talk to the Boys' Club. From him she received invitations to hear SNCC's Stokely Carmichael and Rap Brown, and she accepted. She and Laine attended together.

Suddenly, the warm summer was hot.

Detroit police quickly quelled a crowd of 100 Negroes who stoned cars and store windows along a one-half mile stretch of Kercheval on the east side last night.

The disturbance broke out following the arrest of three men who resisted being ticketed for loitering, police said, on Kercheval. . . .

More than 150 policemen, including riot-trained Tactical Mobile Unit officers, arrived minutes after the disturbance began, but not before at least twelve store windows and numerous car windows had been broken.

(The) Police Comissioner . . . said the disturbance was "definitely not a racial incident."

Six persons were arrested . . . three are reported members of "a militant, extremist organization," the Afro-American Youth Movement. . . . (W. Paul Neal Jr. (byline) *The Detroit News*, August 10, 1966).

Police had put a watch on the A A Y M headquarters. . . . The drab store front, with its painted window and black power symbol on the glass, had been a source of concern. . . . (The next night police reported) "fire-bomb thrown into building, drugstore, burning good" . . . "busting out all the windows, fire trucks can't get through, fire going pretty good, stoning business places, calling for more help. . . ."

(Later) "This thing had no citizen support" (the Police Commissioner) said. "It was only a matter of time until we picked up the ringleaders. . . ."

(He) assessed the damage. Broken windows, damaged cars, four injured policemen, eighteen injured civilians, some $500,000 in overtime pay for police.

"It could have been worse," he said.

For (the) Negro Chairman of the Fifth Precinct Citizens Committee and the block clubs, the damage was seen in another light, too. "We haven't reached those young people down on Kercheval," he said. "We've got to do it. You can't ignore them just because they live six blocks away. You can't ignore people. We've got to get with them, somehow, some way." (Allan Blanchard, *The Detroit News*, August 14, 1966)

At Mom and Tots during those three days in August, the staff continued their work. But there were fewer children in day care, and fewer prenatal patients. The obstetrician did not come; neither did Planned Parenthood's Mrs. McGovern, so Mom and Tots drove the patients to their downtown clinic. Civil unrest does not stop ovulation.

Tommie Sanderson came in to say he was sorry that a brick had made a hole, only a little one, in the Mom and Tots window.

Mrs. Vasiloff was busy ordering new windows for most of her buildings.

Her son had given the keys of the second-floor clinic to men in police uniforms and plain clothes. They returned the keys after making duplicates. They watched the A A Y M storefront at night through the clinic windows. This was not discovered until after the disturbances were past.

Laine was angry at the system. She was incisive. Luke did not like her working at Mom and Tots. "There's nothing wrong with you," she said, "but you're white." She would continue to work with the girls, and in the neighborhood, but not as a representative of the Center. She would use the Center only as a resource.

Luke and Wilson and Abraham had been arrested for "inciting to riot" and were released on a total of $420 bond.[1]

The Negro newspaper, a weekly, viewed the incident.

Officials were fully aware ahead of time of conditions that led to incidents on the Eastside last week. But they chose to ignore them, just as they are choosing to ignore the real problems now, looking only for a scapegoat in the AAYM rather than examining the real problems which cause a group like the AAYM to exist. . . . How can we condone Molotov Cocktails (fire bombs)? But the closer you are to facing the day to day humiliations of police who won't let you stand on your own corners when there is nowhere else to go, of shopkeepers who call you "boy," of teachers who read newspapers in class because they think you're too dumb to learn because you're black, the closer you feel to the boy who heaves one.

And, black or white, the farther away you are from such a situation as exists on Kercheval, the more indignant you become at "agitators."

The real criminals are not the four youths who are accused of "inciting a riot," but the Mayor, the CCR (Detroit Commission on Community Relations), the Police, exploiting shopkeepers, biased teachers, the white paper which did not tell it like it was to the white community, the poverty program officials who didn't set up a program in the Kercheval area, which they acknowledge as one of the worst in the city and who established the nearest community action center miles from there, and members of the Negro middle class who want no part of their brothers jammed into the ghettos.

The city rests peacefully tonight. The "agitators" are caught, and Detroit can go back to its "excellent race relations." Or can it? (Editorial, *The Michigan Chronicle,* August 20, 1966)

They quoted an AAYM member.

"It's not just the police. It's the overpricing, the insults from Whitey. And that TMU (Tactical Mobile Unit). They call it for crime control. Hell, it's a riot squad, a Gestapo, the storm troopers. You don't need a riot force if everything is as good as they are saying." (Carol Schmidt and Jimmy Tinker, *The Michigan Chronicle,* August 20, 1966)

And they interviewed Luke Pride.

"Now we see what power means . . . self-defense. It means making white merchants toe the line on overcharging. It means the dull, day-to-day organizing, not toward getting a house torn down but toward electing a Prosecuting Attorney, not dealing with a policeman who knocks you upside the head, but getting a good force in that won't do it in the first place. It means not integrating schools, but moving to remove the conditions that prevent quality education."
(Ibid.)

The Center heard with foreboding the quarrelsome voices within its own walls; the angry sounds and actions of aroused youth on the street corners; and the tense precautions of law enforcement officers.

And there were other threatening voices, the anonymous voices of health and welfare institutions:

Sorry, we know they didn't get the service they should have, but it wasn't our fault; after all, it was their community that caused the disturbance.

Sorry, we can't help Mom and Tots anymore. We won't have anything to do with any part of this poverty program; we don't like the way the higher-ups are running it. This has nothing to do with you though. . . .

Sorry, we can't take any more appointments for this patient— she's already missed four.

Our organization must have a letter covering each patient referred to us for assistance, giving us their income and expenditures, *in detail.*

We are not set up to subsidize people who are living "high on the hog" by accumulating luxury items on credit and consequently do not have enough funds to cover the cost of medication. There are too many people in this city who are *really* having a struggle to keep a roof over their heads, food in their mouths, and medicine to keep them alive. . . .

We've got to get rid of the tiny pieces. . . . Mom and Tots will have to be absorbed in some other program. . . . The decision was made two or three months ago. . . .

The romance of citizen participation is over.

Actually, we're very proud of that little Center, and we're behind it, but we can't re-fund the program as long as alternative funding exists. . . .

We can't fund the whole thing, let me read you the federal legislation that covers us. . . .

We can't fund you for birth control—our Board you know. . . .

I can't decide it; that is for Washington and Lansing to decide.

If we cooperate, we'd better get good press coverage. . . .

Our hesitation doesn't dilute our endorsement of the concept in principle. . . .

It has a negative image in that location. . . . It doesn't reflect the quality we desire for a medical image. . . .

I would not want to be in a position to judge the adequacy of the whole building. I'm concerned only with quality control of patient care. . . .

The supervision of quality medical care and nursing care needs medical direction.

I cannot see how that building can meet standards of quality. . . . Consider the patients' impressions.

It's too small—we need a facility that can take care of at least 30,000 people. . . .

Is it safe? . . .

It has only a provisional license for day care. . . .[2]

They have teenagers taking care of teenagers.

It's rat infested. . . .

Centers aren't set up for Poles or Italians, why for Negroes? . . .

People are being used. . . .

You'll increasingly have a problem of getting funds with this image.

This is the paradox of a poor area with poor facilities and poor standards—you can't bring in quality care to improve it. . . .

Service alone is not enough without giving these people a chance to improve themselves . . . they need another physical plant . . . one that is an enticement to them. . . .

These people ought to go away from their neighborhood so they can see how other people live—that's the only way they'll want to get out of their poverty. . . .

I cannot go further in recommending funding of any project in that building . . . no matter what the dynamic is there; no health agency can endorse a substandard program. . . .

Would you consider an alternative. . . . Since there are no adequate buildings in the area, why not move the clinic to another area and leave the day care in the storefront?

These people need to act responsibly if they want to be involved. . . . They can't have everything there their own way. . . . You can't do everything they tell you. . . . Leave them alone. . . . There's no need to stir them up again next summer. . . .

If social problems and cultural enrichment are the concern, then this means some other source of funds; under no circumstances could health funds be used. . . .

This is poor medical education for these people. . . . We should teach them to go to proper medical facilities. . . . If we make it too easy for them, they'll never learn to go where they can get proper medical care. . . .

I'm an administrator, a businessman . . . the concept of Mom and Tots is irrelevant to me. . . . I'm concerned about supplies and accounting, and how much this is going to cost us. . . .

Personally, I don't feel this program would benefit us that much . . . after all, we are a professional institution. . . . However, some cooperative arrangement might be possible if there was no money involved on our part. . . .

Why can't you keep this out of the press until negotiations are over?

The voices continued to fall, heavy sounds, repeating themselves, and not hearing themselves, throughout meeting after meeting.

The press spoke.

December 31 may mark the end of the Mom and Tots Center . . . because of cutbacks in poverty program funds and difficulty in unraveling red tape. . . .

In its first nine months of existence the Center spent just $25,000 to provide all its services and to renovate the storefront building it occupies.

Two other agencies have expressed interest in helping to support Mom and Tots. . . . They are the MIC (Maternity and Infant Care) Project and Project PRESCAD (Preschool, School and Adolescent)[3]. . . . However, support from these agencies will be delayed until budget amendments can be approved in Washington. . . . This will require a minimum of three months.

The Mayor's Committee for Total Action Against Poverty (TAP) (has been) appealed to for an extension of its support. A meeting is scheduled. . . . (Colleen O'Brien, *The Detroit Free Press,* December 13, 1966)

(The) deputy director of TAP told the Visiting Nurse Association at a meeting Tuesday at TAP headquarters, that TAP no longer can support the community health center. . . . Mom and Tots is one project that has to go because it is not included in the revised TAP guidelines.

A meeting with United Community Services . . . has been scheduled for Wednesday. The VNA, which administers the Center, is a Torch Drive (United Community Services) agency. (C. O'Brien, *The Detroit Free Press,* December 14, 1966)

The fate of Mom and Tots . . . is in the hands of the Central Budget Committee of United Community Services. . . . If UCS decides to bridge the gap, the Center can operate while negotiations with other federally-funded projects are carried out. . . . (C. O'Brien, *The Detroit Free Press,* December 15, 1966)

The grandeur of American world power hears "with a disdainful smile the short and simple annals of the poor."

So, to finance the war in Viet-

nam, the funds to fight another war, closer to home, have been cut by $4 million in Detroit. It is the poor who pay for our misdirected vision of world leadership. One of the first to pay is the Mom and Tots Center, . . . in the heart of urban poverty and last summer's urban unrest. . . . (Editorial, *The Detroit Free Press,* December 16, 1966)

. . . a neighborhood center practically fashioned with their own hands, which more than adequately provides the help and support so many of them desperately need, is about to close its doors because the Federal funds under which it operates have been cut off due to mounting costs of the Vietnam conflict. . . . (*The Michigan Chronicle,* January 28, 1967)

The Mom and Tots Center . . . a pilot project in preventive health care, got a stay of execution. . . . Its rescuer— temporary—is the Central Budget Committee of USC, which has allocated $24,000 to the Center for not more than a six-month period.

(The) director of USC said that with this fund the Center can carry on . . . while it negotiates for possible federal funds. If these are not obtainable, the program will be phased out. . . . (*The Detroit Free Press,* December 20, 1966)

The Mom and Tots Center may become a permanent establishment if current negotiations with Detroit Memorial Hospital are successful.

(The Hospital may be willing) to accept the medical—but not financial—responsibility. The directors of two federally funded public health projects (MIC and PRESCAD) . . . expressed interest in picking up the Center, but nothing came of it. . . . (C. O'Brien, *The Detroit Free Press*, February 17, 1967)

With the decision* by Detroit Memorial Hospital last week to accept medical responsibility for the Mom and Tots Center, part of the problems were over. . . .

To date, no permanent arrangements (for funds) have been made. (C. O'Brien, *The*

Detroit Free Press, April 17, 1967)

Mr. Speaker, the story of an interesting and apparently effective antipoverty project appeared in *The Detroit Free Press* of December 8, 1966. . . . The subject of the article is the Mom and Tots Center, an antipoverty storefront outpost in Detroit. . . . Its purpose is to provide a variety of health services to low-income residents of the area. . . .

Mr. Speaker, . . . I commend the *Free Press* article to the attention of our colleagues and ask that it be printed at this point in the Record. . . . (Congressman James O'Hara of Michigan, *U.S. Congressional Record, House of Representatives,* February 6, 1967, p. H 1052).

* Three weeks later, this decision was reversed, and the prenatal program was cancelled completely.

But such a commendation, even by the House, would be an epitaph if the Center could not find a way to apply for federal funds.

On
the
inside

and the outside, the destructive
forces were always present, and I was sometimes at a loss to know
how to deal with them all at the same time.

No matter how good the Center appeared to those outside
it, it would lose its vitality if those who worked in it did not learn
to appreciate the different viewpoints among themselves. Felecia,
who in her apparent simplicity could often cut through jargon and
get to the core of the matter, said it for the staff: in evaluating
their programs, they needed first to look at themselves. With sen-
sitivity, Felecia would often speak for herself, about herself. Then
the others followed.

Increasingly, the very process of talking not only gave
them direction, but also provided an atmosphere in which
their attempts at solution could be carried out. The satisfactions
gained through talking, being listened to by each other, and trying
things mutually agreed to, encouraged more group effort.

Moving Ada to the second floor brought about a marked
change in her demeanor. It was a dramatic reminder to me of how
structure, the physical environment, limits or allows the expression of human potential, and how people can, if they will, shape

circumstances to make them permissive of human expression.

Outside the Center there were potentially stifling threats. There were the obvious forces of destruction and physical violence, described in such different tones by the white and Negro press. Apparently, A C M E (now The Afro-American Youth Movement) placed no blame on the Center when I sent word to them that without my knowledge the police, or men who appeared to be police, were using the Center at night for their watch. My thinking was the Center would be safer if they knew the truth over which we had no control. The fact that we had no control over the police was a distressing new experience for me.

The other kind of threat came from long-established health institutions. Their voices could be as damaging to health as firebombs, as destructive of health care as the occupation of private premises by police is to law and order. Their pronouncements revealed much about what they stood for: punitive in tone, competitive, self-protecting, concerned with surface qualities and with parts of people, seeking to have people fit the "system" rather than the reverse, viewing "responsible action" as compliance with their rules.

As I noted before, the meaning of the Mom and Tots story in the professional world will await another telling. It is enough to say here that before its first year was over the Center lost its operating grant from OEO. And, it was informed by officials responsible for prenatal care services that regardless of finances in 1967, the Center's prenatal program would be cancelled.

It was a painful irony to know that at the very moment that Mom and Tots was going on record in the Congress as a successful OEO (poverty) program, the funds for its survival were being withdrawn by OEO.

I could not help thinking how the Center's struggle to survive paralleled a fact of life in the existence of poor people; that continual concern over physical necessities often crowds out the more intangible aspects of human wholeness. I wondered whether this would happen to the Center during the six months it was given to find money to go on. Would I be so intent on finding funds and on retaining a prenatal program that I would not give sufficient energy to the inner life of the Center, the people, without which the money would mean little?

V
In
the
Balance

The world is changing and anyone who thinks he can live alone

is sleeping through a revolution. . . .

MARTIN LUTHER KING
Memphis, Tennessee
March 31, 1968

DON'T LET MOM & TOTS DIE....

Join your neighbors at a meeting on

Sunday February 5, 1967

at 3 P.M. (Hot coffee served)....

A green flier went out to schools and churches and block clubs in the neighborhood. The teens stuffed the envelopes.

Regi organized his Boys' Club members to pass them door-to-door. He would work extra time to pass them himself, without pay. He had already painted over the "funded by TAP" phrase on the Center's sign, even in January weather.

Felecia washed all the curtains. Mrs. Watkins took them home to iron. Felecia's husband Bernard was home from Viet Nam for good now; he would help, too. She called the "soul music station" for support on the air. She talked to the PTA at Pingree Elementary about the Center's crisis.

Mertus contacted the state senator whose campaign she'd worked on. She thought they ought to have the patients speak at the meeting. She would be willing to lead it. No, she couldn't start working full time; if she did, she'd lose her ADC grant and then if the Center closed, she would have a long, hard time getting back on ADC.

Hank's mother had reported the Center's plight to the ADC Mothers Federation to which she belonged.

Ada Dixon and Mrs. Jefferson composed a questionnaire which they sent to all the prenatal patients.

> How do you feel about the services rendered to you at the Mom and Tots Prenatal Clinic?
> Would you recommend the Clinic to others?
> Is this location convenient to you?
> Would you want it changed?
> If so, how? . . .

Mrs. Jefferson had already begun a petition in her neighborhood.

Mary Louise was willing to work more hours—not full time yet. But she would contact her brother-in-law who knew someone in Washington. She knew the editor of the Negro newspaper; they would endorse Sunday's meeting. She also knew someone in the Urban League to whom she'd talk.

Laine called to learn the details. She and Luke had agreed that if Mom and Tots closed, this would be another example of broken promises by the Establishment.

There was a heavy snow February 5. Hazardous driving warnings were out. The day was gray.

Ada and Mrs. Jefferson were at the Center early to prepare coffee, while the boys arranged chairs.

Almost fifty people came. There weren't enough chairs, so they sat on the children's chairs, on Mary Louise's desk, on the piano bench, on the storefront window ledges.

Several prenatal patients came; four called later and said they couldn't come in the snow. Some day-care mothers came. Mr. and Mrs. Ford from Pingree PTA; their son Willie was on the day-care waiting list. Mr. and Mrs. Cross, a young white couple new in the neighborhood. Mrs. George, the practical nurse. And CESSA, Churches on the East Side for Social Action, a new interfaith group of about twenty-five local churches; Rev. Clay Shaw, Rev. Keith Hill, Father Tom Riley stood at the back; several laymen from their congregations sat among the others.

By 3:30, Mertus hadn't arrived. Mrs. Jefferson thought it was time to begin. She told the gathering that the Center not only served the neighborhood with clinic and day care and transportation, but it also was a place to keep the kids off the street. She introduced the staff.

The group heard the story of the sudden loss of funds for Mom and Tots, that it now had five months in which to find a permanent source of support, that the prenatal clinic would very likely be discontinued even if funds were found, and they were told that the Center wanted to be what the neighborhood wanted it to be.

One mother stood up. "You mean if it goes on, we could have a all-day day-care program? Well, I'd be willing to take a petition to my neighbors to sign. . . ."

Other women and men joined in agreement. Ada Dixon dashed upstairs to type out petitions, as Mertus came in the door clutching the sore throat that had made her late.

Rev. Shaw said his church across the street, Allan Temple, would be happy to share its parking lot as a playground, and help with renovations. He'd like to bring the problem to the whole CESSA Executive Board next week. "Look's like we might have to loosen a few stiff shirts!" he said.

Hand-clapping and "Amens" accompanied his speech. Mrs. Watkins led the "Amens."

One by one, the prenatal patients stood up and said why they wanted a prenatal clinic.

> There isn't any hours of waiting and you get the very best attention. . . .

> The location of the clinic is convenient for me. It helps me to keep my appointments. . . .

> I can bring my children if I don't have no one to watch them. . . .

> They make you feel like you're somebody. . . .

One very pregnant mother suggested that all the patients get together to write out their opinions of the clinic; then maybe this would convince the health officials and doctors who did not want Mom and Tots to have a prenatal clinic. Six women each took the names of five patients; they would get together for a party in two weeks and write down their opinions.

A dozen people took petitions from Ada Dixon. Rev. Hill would speak to the local junior high-school Teacher-Community Committee. Another mother volunteered to talk to the parents at a neighboring school. . . .

Together they were caught up in the impulse to respond to the nameless forces that would constrict and stifle.

Most kept their promises.

Strategy meetings were held with and among churchmen and school women.

CESSA wrote letters:

> Frankly, we are extremely disturbed over this. . . . A number

of congregations in CESSA are located near the Center and we have seen the worth of the services being performed there. We simply cannot understand this lack of cooperation on (your) part, when (these) services are needed in the area and can be offered at the Center which is an asset for the development of the area as a whole. . . .

CESSA sent a delegation to influential physicians.

People signed petitions and these were turned in and forwarded to those in authority.

Patients filled out the questionnaires and half of these were mailed back to the Center.

Fourteen of the prenatal patients met at the Center for an early afternoon party. Mrs. Watkins and Felecia served coffee and oatmeal cookies.

Felecia chattered about the day-care children. Mrs. Watkins explained how the young ones would eat liver if it were ground up into Sloppy Joe's, with hamburger and tomatoes and carrots.

Some mothers thought they'd like to see what the children were fed, to give them ideas for home. Some wondered about how you get your child to do what he's supposed to do without "whippin' " him all the time. Some worried about questions on sex. . . . Couldn't they meet again and talk more about these things? So began the Mothers Club.

Felecia talked about the dream of an all-day day-care program. But it would be awfully expensive.

"Well I'd be willing to pay something. . . ."

They exchanged suggestions about what would be a fair fee. Then one said, "Each mother could pay what she earns in an hour for the day. That be fair. . . ."

Nonworking mothers?

"They could give time like they do now."

They began to dream together. A playground. An enlarged Center. A Center station wagon. . . .

Felecia brought them back. "But ladies, today, we got to do something about this here prenatal clinic. . . ."

Eventually, they wrote down their thoughts:

I like the service very much. There is no long waiting period to see the doctor or to get the medicine he perscribes. . . .

There are different things you should know on the wall pin on a board. . . .

It is closer to me. The doctor and nurses are nice. They understand you. I think very highly about the Clinic because of the peoples that's wait on you. Plus it is not crowded.

They is very nice and polite every time I go up to the Clinic. . . .

The employee that work here is very nice and they try to help you the best they can. . . .

Their thoughts went to those in authority.

But their voices were ignored.

The search for funds went on. Public resources, for physical health, for mental health, for poverty, for welfare, for child care. Private foundations, in Michigan, in New York, in Massachusetts.

The Center continued to struggle with its internal conflicts.

Mertus summarized with thoroughness the articles in a new journal on children she'd just subscribed to. She had read them all—except the one on sex education—and she would report on them to the others.

"You know, I'm a little upset," she said in private.

She didn't like Mary Louise's "nagging" about organization. She said Mary Louise didn't want to talk about the children enough, only "organization." Mary Louise shouldn't be sitting in on the day-care discussions. Mertus felt she was "being accused of not carrying my share." No, *she* had no feelings against any of *them*.

Mary Louise gave her view privately, too: Mertus always thought she was right; so how could she be corrected? She would never admit to a mistake. But Mary Louise agreed to avoid the day-care discussions.

And Mrs. Watkins said of Mertus, "Don't do no work when

she comes nohow—unless it's somethin' special; don't help set up for lunch; . . . always on that phone; . . . talk too much at quiet time. . . ."

And Felecia complained that Mertus was not going to show them the report Mr. Hughes had drawn up for the VNA on the day-care program. She got a copy from Ada Dixon anyway, and she didn't like it at all. She, Mrs. Watkins, and Ada had read it together. "It ain't so much what he said but the way he said it. . . . He tore down what we been building. . . . He talked about *us* and not the children. . . . I don't like being called names. He can call me 'low-income' if he thinks I am, but not 'low-class'. . . . And Mertus didn't think none of that was so bad. . . ."

A week later, Mertus called the Center. The water pipes had broken and she couldn't come in. Six weeks of uncertainty followed. She lost her babysitter. Kay was "acting-out" in kindergarten and was sent home; a second time; a third time. Two more water pipes broke. Kay didn't want to go back to school; she was "hysterical" when Mertus wanted to leave for work.

Would Mertus like to go to a counselor with Kay? The Center could arrange it.

Mertus came back to work sporadically.

She called again. It was "too hard to face Mrs. Watkins and Felecia. . . ." She didn't want to "rush into counseling. . . ." "I guess I'm not very free at saying what I feel. . . ." She needed time to think.

Vacation time. Sick leave time.

She was called. She preferred taking a leave of absence, indefinitely.

Could she consider junior college? Help with tuition?

No, not now.

At the end of winter, the Center knew that Mertus was on leave of absence, indefinitely.

The staff set up a new day-care schedule. They asked Mrs. Ford—who had become more and more interested in the Center since the February meeting—if she wanted to work as a substitute. She did. Johnnie West would help too. Mrs. Watkins was talking to neighbors; she thought one, Mrs. House, "would make us a real good cook" when we get our new program: "I got faith we will."

Life went on more smoothly, though tentatively, with no realistic hope of funds, but with many plans for a better Center.

Hank would occasionally stop in at the Center using a walker. He was having his legs exercised daily now; the Center paid a neighbor $10 a week to do this under Carol Howard's supervision. He would soon begin training at a vocational rehabilitation center.

Mom and Tots had a new housekeeper, Mrs. Jack, one of Ada's neighbors. She was Hank's replacement. When she was hospitalized for thyroid surgery, her husband and children continued with her evening chores at the Center.

The children, after school hours, wanted to learn to dance. Mary Louise found two high-school seniors, prospective physical education teachers, willing to help. Ralph led a series in calisthenics for the boys, and Terry, Mrs. Queen's daughter, a modern dance series for the girls: coordinating exercises, dance positions, and music, from romanticism to jazz.

One of Johnnie West's new responsibilities was to acquaint mothers in the neighborhood with the Center. She spent a few hours a week visiting in their homes. In a little notebook she wrote what they wanted, or what they wanted to know when she didn't have the answers at hand.

Phone calls came from community agencies asking: What is Mom and Tots? They had difficulty fitting it into familiar categories.

Other calls and letters came asking another question: how can we have something like Mom and Tots? From churches and poverty programs, student health groups, and health professionals, ADC mothers groups and universities, and the Girl Scouts.

Other calls asked: can we tour Mom and Tots? From women's clubs, professional schools, agencies. Almost without exception the answer to this question was "No." In response, some groups said "Don't you want the publicity?" "Don't you need money?" The answer was "Yes, we need money, but No."

One Sunday evening, a pick-up truck, trying to avoid children playing in the alley, swerved and crashed into the window. Ada Dixon heard the news and within an hour had the police and landlord at the Center.

Life went on at Mom and Tots, except in the boarded-up corner.

Mrs. Vasiloff was slow to deal with her share of the repairs. Nor had she tended to other maintenance problems which irritated and interfered with life at the Center. She received a letter from a legal firm.

> . . . We have been informed by the Visiting Nurse Association that there are conditions existing at the subject premises which require immediate correction. Specifically, we refer to a number of repairs, the making of which is your responsibility as lessor of the premises. Furthermore, we understand that you have on many occasions represented to the Visiting Nurse Association that such repairs will be made by you. However, none of the subject repairs have as yet been made by you.
>
> Therefore. . . .
>
> The following repairs, the performance of which you have previously admitted to be your obligation, are to be commenced by you. . . . If said repairs are not made by you. . . . performance thereof will be undertaken by the Visiting Nurse Association and the cost of said repairs will be deducted . . . from the rental payment. . . .

Soon the Center had not only new windows, but workable doors and transoms, toilets and faucets, drains and lights; and two new screen-storm doors, deducted from the rent.

Plans continued to evolve for an enlarged Mom and Tots without any tangible evidence that they would be realized. But Mrs. Watkins kept her faith.

Letters went out to CESSA churches, to block clubs, and to neighborhood groups for a full-time day-care supervisor to lead a ten-hour day-care program; a driver to transport patients in a still nonexistent Center stationwagon; a community worker; a community health nurse, and a contractor to extend the Center into the adjacent storefront and to build a playground.

CESSA talked of hiring a community-organizer who could get to the boys in the Afro-American Youth Movement. Perhaps Mom and Tots could help acquaint him with the neighborhood.

Occasionally, Luke stepped across the street to see Mary Louise. One day he announced that the charges against him from last August's disturbance had been dropped. He spoke to the Boys Club about fighting, about protection for what you love as the only motive for fighting.

AAYM members would come to reiterate their views on birth control to Mary Louise. She listened quietly and responded without antagonizing.

The son of one of the AAYM members, another who had been arrested in August, was enrolled in day care by his mother.

But in late spring, much of the money coming from white supporters of AAYM disappeared, principally because certain of the white supporters left the Detroit area. AAYM headquarters looked deserted.

That spring, 1967, the Center received an award for improving police-community relations from the Fifth Precinct Citizen-Police Community Organization. The CPCO membership was composed of block clubs and churches, and the remnants of the old Eastside Improvement Association. It had formed the previous summer, shortly before August.

"Lord have mercy!" said Mrs. Watkins in a mixture of disbelief and delight that the Center should receive such an award.

From the time that the news of Mom and Tots' impending collapse was published, letters and phone calls crisscrossed the country. Detroit to San Francisco, to Chicago, to New York, to Washington, D.C.

Slowly, a network of communication formed, then developed into a cushion in support of the Center. The network extended from the local maneuverings of liberal suburbanite women and VNA board members, nurse-educators and students, clergy and judges, professors and deans, nurses and physicians, to state senators and representatives and health officials, to U.S. congressmen and senators, to the National offices of Health, Education, and Welfare, and to the Office of Economic Opportunity.

Negro nurses had talked to Negro physicians who had found two Negro hospitals that wanted to be "involved in the community." They would cooperate with Mom and Tots in a new prenatal clinic and maternity service.

In late spring, a phone call came from Detroit poverty headquarters, TAP. Would Mom and Tots come to pick up an application for OEO funds?

Three weeks later, another phone call came from TAP headquarters. Mom and Tots would be getting OEO funds, no one knew how much.

"Have mercy! I told you we was gonna get it somehow," said Mrs. Watkins.

Whatever the amount, it was enough to hold another Sunday afternoon meeting. The pink flier read:

HELP MOM & TOTS GROW
We need your
ideas, suggestions, muscles,
and skills. . . .

Committees, colors, clinic times were chosen.

The funding was officially announced two months later:

The Mom and Tots Center will cease its hand-to-mouth existence and begin an expansion of services immediately because of a new grant awarded by the U.S. Office of Economic Opportunity.

The $42,000 grant, to be spent over the next seven

months, was announced this week by Sen. Philip A. Hart.

(However), Money for improvements (necessary to meet state licensing requirements) was not included in the grant. . . . (C. O'Brien, *The Detroit Free Press,* July 13, 1967)

The additional $15,000 needed for renovations to meet licensing requirements for the new day-care program, playground, and station wagon bus came from the new friends of Mom and Tots. From individuals and families in amounts from $2 to $200. From groups, churches, and private boards and clubs, in $500 to $4000 gifts.

The cushion which had saved the Center would continue to help sustain it.

But no cushion, no encapsulating medium from outside the neighborhood, could have protected the Center from what was to come July 23, 1967: a historic date for Detroit and for the American city.

For
myself,
in the

winter of 1967, I was ready to
stop the struggle. I was tired. I hurt, in body and soul. And what
made the weight heavier was that I knew the truth of what was
told me: if I stopped even to rest there would be no one on the
professional side to carry on.

In a real sense, the Center carried me. I had kept the staff
informed of every meeting and action taken by the political and
health hierarchies affecting the Center. They probably had a better understanding of the politics of health than many of my professional colleagues. There seemed to be no question in their
minds that the Center would fight, and not only fight, but win—
bless Mrs. Watkins for her faithful fatalism. Without my knowledge they had begun various tactics around their own homes and
had been keeping the patient-groups and other Center people informed of what was happening.

I told them that it was no longer enough that they and I
wanted the Center to continue, or that the VNA wanted it to go
on; the people in the neighborhood had to want it enough to do

something about keeping it. Thus came the decision to call the February meeting.

It was a lively and vocal crowd that packed the Center on that snowy Sunday. Many of the people did not know me. I was introduced as one of the staff, one who could give more details on the financial and prenatal clinic situation. There was little awareness, if any, of what the VNA was, or that it was the sponsoring agency for the Center. I was careful not to suggest any particular course of action. My hope was that the beginnings of a governing board from the neighborhood would form, one that could be either ancillary to or independent of the VNA Board of Trustees, with perhaps representatives from the VNA, from the Center's staff, from the patients, and from neighborhood individuals and groups. My thinking was based on two considerations. First, since most official health structures in the City were disavowing the Center in fact if not in concept, this augured poorly for having traditional health care services at the Center in the near future. Thus, the neighborhood could more readily give it a neighborhood day-care-recreation focus than a neighborhood health-care focus. Second, such a board, acting in interdependence with the VNA, or choosing to be independent eventually, would represent another step toward achieving a kind of ideal in terms of the basic concept of health implicit in the Mom and Tots Center. The VNA, now actively involved in the struggle to save the Center, was willing to consider this move and to finance the necessary legal procedures if it evolved.

However, the kinds of suggestions for action which were made at that Sunday meeting pertained directly to the immediate crisis and were of an ad hoc nature. I asked the group what they wanted the Center to be like in the future, if it continued. As usual, full-time day care was talked about most. Without leads from the group, I knew it would be meaningless for me to suggest the idea of a neighborhood board. Besides, the staff had decided that the Center should not pursue the idea unless or until there were clear indications that people wanted it.

Nevertheless, the primary purpose of the meeting, to discern whether the Center, in their minds, was worth fighting for, was accomplished. The efforts by neighborhood people on behalf of the Center made it a part of their community. The staff at the Center showed a degree of initiative that I had not seen before. I learned later that they had decided to avoid taking their problems to me, to work them out among themselves, so that I could attend to the worrisome task of money-hunting.

There was no real hope of finding sufficient funds. Mom and Tots as an entity simply did not fit into any existing funding categories. But one thing became clear to me after that February meeting: if we were going to continue, the new Center ought to be what people had been wanting for so long. It should have a bigger and longer day-care program, a full-time transportation service, a playground, and a recreation area especially for older children. So I rewrote the grant proposal accordingly.

Unfortunately, community attempts to confront the decision-makers in the world of health-politics were even less effective than mine in concert with the VNA. The CESSA delegation, for instance, was completely disregarded, and their efforts very likely produced a greater resistance among the health professionals in high places. Their efforts were not wasted, however, in terms of establishing solidarity between the Center and the neighborhood. Thus, at the time, my role as intermediary was an essential one.

I also explained the meaning of the Center to segments of the professional and lay worlds, since many people became interested because of or as a result of the publicity the Center was receiving. But their direct efforts also failed to move the existing power structure—the policy-makers and the sources of health funds.

It was only when Washington became aware of what was happening via elected officials who had been informed by certain well-to-do women who were active as board members of community agencies or behind the scenes in political campaigns, as well as by a few professional people, that local decision-makers felt constrained to save the Center.

Thus, the really influential ones who made possible the financial and structural supports needed for the Center—a controversial and nontraditional undertaking—were members of the white and Negro affluent classes. Both groups as stereotypes, and especially its nonemployed women, are often labeled conservative and narrow, uncaring about the rest of society, tenacious of the status quo. Whether the tides of change are bringing a new breed of affluent people, black and white, whether my perceptions of them as individuals—who are, of course, not just members of gross categories—are sharper, or both, I do not know. But they do exist. And they have the power and will to act in the interests of the wholeness of society.

As the Center became known, many requests were made to visit it. My thinking was that the general question of observers coming from outside the neighborhood had to be answered in terms of the focus of the Mom and Tots Center. If the Center were to focus on the interests and needs of neighborhood people and to try to act in accordance with their wishes, it could not at the same time give *priority* to the interests and needs of outside agencies—whether service agencies, educational institutions, or clubs of good will.

So, when health professionals were permitted to visit, they came as participants, not observers, preferably without uniform; they came as listeners and learners. Priority was given to Black visitors, whose presence was least disruptive of the Center's spontaneity and informality.

In other words, I sought to convey to health professionals that the V N A was a guest in the neighborhood and at the Center. Therefore, the V N A was not in a position to invite other outsiders to come in without the permission, and much less without the invitation, of the people there.

The inner life of the Center moved in spite of, or perhaps because of, its external predicament. I saw no reason not to try whatever the staff or various groups wanted. If the Center were to end on July 1, it would at least have been as much as it could have been.

The staff weathered Mertus' absence very well. In a sense I am sure they were relieved, since they could never see her potential as clearly as her limitations; but perhaps she could not either. I personally was disappointed that we could not find a way for her to remain and I tried to leave a path open for her to return in the future. She did contact the Center three times in the following year, each time in connection with job applications.

And the staff exploded healthfully about Mr. Hughes's report. Later, they confronted him with their objections. He changed certain terminology, such as "lower-class" to "low-income," and omitted certain generalizations such as those concerning their feelings toward men. They approved the report before it was officially submitted to the VNA.

Through the months of crisis the Center revealed a certain amount of independence, as well as the extent of dependence on the world outside. In a broader sense our activities demonstrated the interdependence of ALL people, poor and affluent, professionals and laymen, black and white. But that interdependency would be dramatized far more vividly in the next crisis, only days away.

VI
Convulsion

We must learn to live together as brothers or we will perish together as fools. . . . Racial injustice is still the black man's burden and the white man's shame. . . . The government must certainly share the guilt, the individual must share the guilt and even the church must share the guilt.

MARTIN LUTHER KING
Memphis, Tennessee
March 31, 1968

White society is deeply implicated in the ghetto. White institutions created it, white institutions maintain it, and white society condones it. . . .

President's National Advisory
Commission on Civil Disorder
February, 1968

July 23, 1967:

The city burns.
Fires dot ghetto neighborhoods.
Smoke mounts on the horizon.
Flames spread to stores, houses, churches.

On the streets young people
Saunter up to the store windows at which they once window-
    shopped and eyed the contents with envy.
They enter through casements broken by rioters and help
    themselves.
They lug TV's, appliances, hosiery, candy.
They push carts and pull wagons full of goods.
Children grin and run.

As night comes you can hear sounds not common for a Sunday
    night in July:
Cracks that echo and ricochet,
Sirens,
The roar of cars,
The ring of laughter,
The tenseness of the newscasters.

Police patrol, four in a car;
Their rifles pointed out the windows;
Their helmets strapped tight.

The night stays lit by
Streetlights,
Floodlights,
Police beams,
And flames.[1]

The riot which began on a Sunday morning on the north-
west side spread quickly throughout the core of the city. During the first three days, the Mom and Tots staff kept each
other informed about the fate of the Center via a phone chain.

By midnight Sunday, Ada Dixon reported, threatening
crowds were gathering in the neighborhood. Within two hours
the burnings began on Kercheval.

At daylight the next morning, Mrs. Watkins sent her
husband to Kercheval, two blocks away. The laundromat, the

drugstore, the dimestore, were looted. National Guard troops were not allowing anyone to leave for work. The fires continued. Mom and Tots was not touched.

That afternoon Ada learned from the postman that the dry cleaner near the Center was looted. More fires burned.

By eight that night the supermarket was looted and the drugstore and hardware store were burning.

On the morning of the third day, Mrs. Jack had her husband get the news on Kercheval. A fourteen-year-old had been shot; a fireman was killed; most stores were damaged; looting was spreading. But the Center was safe.

Later that morning, Luke and Laine, and then the new organizer hired by CESSA, Dan Frank, spoke to Mary Louise. They said that Mom and Tots remained, that someone had written "B" (for "Soul Brother")[2] on the window.

In the afternoon, Mrs. Ford's husband checked on the Center. She proudly reported, "Mom and Tots stands out like a sore thumb" among the gutted buildings.

The Mayor and Governor, on Tuesday night, encouraged Detroiters to return to work the next day. Via the phone chain, the staff, with some apprehension, agreed to meet at the Center the next morning. Mary Louise would give up her vacation in the crisis.

The staff members were talking to their neighbors, trying to find out how the Center could be most helpful. Mary Louise attended a CESSA meeting for the same reason. Dan Frank asked to use the Center's newly acquired storefront next door for food distribution and a press conference.

Wednesday morning, after a quick meeting around the kitchen table, the staff decided. "We should be what we are." Mom and Tots would continue its activities and would cooperate with CESSA and ESVID, the East Side Voice of Independent Detroit, Dan Frank's new group.[3] But Ada was suspicious of Dan Frank; she thought he condoned the riot. She was reluctant to allow the storefront to be used for food distribution because looters might break in at night.

Nevertheless, the Center followed its chosen course.

It was "business as usual"—but not really. Although children were in day care, they belonged to women waiting in the food line. They were not the regular day-care youngsters, some of whose mothers were afraid to bring them. Although the Planned Parenthood Clinic was in session, Johnnie West was packing donated baby food for distribution in between leading group discussions with the patients.

The day-care staff prepared breakfast for a tired pregnant woman in the food line. They offered a cold drink to the elderly, some of whom waited three to four hours for their bag of groceries. Carloads of food, milk, vitamins, formula, soap, diapers arrived. The Center's teens and mothers, the ministers and priests of CESSA, the bearded members of ESVID together distributed the donations. Even one of Pete Collins Jackson's sons helped. "It went well—not smoothly, but well," said Mary Louise, as food for 1277 adults and children was given away.

Outside, prisoners, closely watched by National Guardsmen, shoveled glass and debris from the streets, as the clean-up process began. Leaflets were circulated, such as one describing the Black Star Cooperative:

> . . . we have come together. We believe that by combining our bodies, our minds and our resources, we will increase our strength a thousand-fold, whatever our number be, and in this manner, we will begin the long and joyful task of rebuilding ourselves, our families and our communities.

> We intend to:

> 1. Establish a cooperative housing corporation designed to bring us together in one place, so that we may support one another in our endeavors and free a larger portion of our resources for the task at hand.

> 2. Combine our resources for the establishment of various business enterprises in our community.

> 3. Combine our resources to gain greater influence and control over the political and social life of our community.[4]

Mrs. Vasiloff came, cautiously inspecting the damage to

her property. She had received threatening phone calls, calling her "white trash."

The immediate need had been food, since virtually all neighborhood markets had been gutted. Within a few days, food supplies were about as accessible as they had been prior to the riot.

The other problems, housing, economic limitations, child care facilities, ready transportation were no different in the east side ghetto from what they had been before the riot. The only difference perhaps was that now everybody knew that everybody knew about them.[5]

The white press searched for causes:	The Negro press searched for causes:
Is it possible that agitators employed some devious device to provoke police to raid the after-hours hangouts? (which precipitated the riot). . . . A number of police and military officials are convinced that this was the work of well-trained groups, possibly belonging to a national antiwhite conspiratorial organization. . . .	The immediate problem at hand could have been handled. . . . editor-general manager of the Michigan Chronicle was on the scene. He saw the hoodlums begin their looting and their burning. He saw the police stand as if helpless. Right at this point the situation could have been quelled. . . . But he still wonders if early in the day, "Did the police just write off 12th Street?" (where the riot began). . . . The mayor . . . and Police Commissioner . . . felt that the thing would stop there. . . .
"We tried to sweep the streets like we did last summer" (the Police Commissioner) said, "But it didn't work. I still think we were right. I'm convinced that it would have grown bigger sooner if we had used more force. There was really no way to put it down without a standing army. . . ."	

(The Mayor) "There is a huge section of our society that is not really part of it. The people feel left out and get committed to complete lawlessness at the slightest excuse."

(The Governor's) assessment is . . . that it was primarily the work of the "lawless and criminal elements."

As it is almost everywhere in America today, the Negro leadership is deeply divided in Detroit. The division is complex. There are the leaders the whites will listen to and those the new breed of militant young Negroes will listen to. It boils down to the Black Power advocates and (those) who want to pursue peaceful but progressive policies. . . . (Tom Joyce, "Anatomy of Detroit Rioting," *The Detroit News,* July 30, 1967)

. . . Frustrations, despair, this feeling of not being wanted, no place to go, broke loose . . . our people needed . . . to be rescued from the entrapment of employment restrictions, of what they felt were exploitation from the landlords, the storeowners, the police, the city officials. . . .

We can't allow our city to be taken over by lawless hoodlums . . . we have to . . . go to work and get that little fellow to know that this is his city too. And he can't gain anything by destroying it.

Our leaders knew that trouble was upon us. . . . Direct action by our organization was stymied by internecine warfare, power struggle for recognition and personal aggrandizement. "Young Turks" fought the "Old Guard," the extremists fought the moderates, the professionals fought the unionists . . . civil rights organizations had done little to get at the basic problems that have undermined the minds, the morals of our community for the past 20 years. (Editorial, *The Michigan Chronicle,* July 29, 1967)

At a press conference, Dan Frank interpreted the riot:

What is necessary is that we understand the people and then maybe we can understand the rebellion. It is said that the burning and looting were indiscriminate. This was not true. The Mom and Tots Center was not touched during the rebellion, though buildings on both sides were burned and gutted. Why?

Because black folks said: "These are good people. We know them and they know us. They work with us, not on us like one works on a machine, or a piece of wood. They care for us. We know we can stop in and they'll help us when we ask them things. They ask us to make decisions on how to run the place. They treat us like first-class humans because we are first-class humans. They have respect for us and we respect them."

They were not burned.
(C. O'Brien, *The Detroit Free Press*, July 30, 1967)

I
watched
the

city burn. The days of fire, which changed the climate of Detroit if little else, had surrealist qualities. It was at once a mass involvement in the urban tragedy and a mass depersonalization, as though you were watching yourself through it all but could not believe you were part of what was happening, victim and perpetrator, ally and enemy.

It was like an incident that occurred not far from Twelfth Street in an apartment building known as a "gem in the manure pile," one of the few comfortable living places in that part of the city. On an afternoon during the peak of the riot, a Negro mother rushed down a carpeted hall of the building to an elevator with her preschool child. He was wearing his baseball cap and clutched his toy fishing rod. She carried a bag of toys. She looked harried.

At the same time, three responsible young white women stepped out of their apartment. One asked the mother, "You're leaving the building?"

"Yes," said the Negro. "Isn't it awful?"

Her little boy said to them, "I like the big fire. . . . I mean. . . . I like the big fire engines." He somehow knew enough not to say he liked the *fires*.

One of the white women, wearing a pair of binoculars, asked her Negro neighbor, "Can we help you?"

"Well. . . ." The Negro hesitated. "There are just two more bags. . . . I have to go back. . . ."

"Let us carry them for you." Two of the white women, the one with the binoculars, and another, holding a camera, escorted the Negro back to her apartment, and each brought out a bag.

The group walked quickly to the elevator. The Negro continued, "Isn't it awful, isn't it *awful?*" The white women agreed.

Only the mother and child entered the elevator. The pair with binoculars and camera laid the bags on the elevator floor, stepped back out, and one of them pressed "Lobby" on the push-button panel.

"Oh," said the Negro, "aren't you going down too?"

"Oh no," said one of the others, "we're going up to the roof to see if we can get some pictures."

Just then I could say nothing, as I saw myself and my two friends contributing to the terrible irony of the situation. And how many others were there like us, in their homes watching the burning on their TV sets?

Watching the flames, smelling the smoke from my relatively safe vantage point high above Twelfth Street, confined by the curfew, there was much time to think. But I could not. I could only feel the greatest sadness I had ever felt up to that time. The tears seemed useless, too.

Literally throughout the first days and nights of the rioting, the Mom and Tots staff kept a watch on the Center and kept me informed by phone about what was happening on Kercheval. I waited for the message that said it was burning. I thought it would burn, if not by intention, then surely by accident, or that at the least it would be damaged. And how could we begin all over again?

But there was no damage. The curfew was lifted. And regardless of uncertainties and advice to the contrary, it was time to act. That the Center remained when all the storefronts for blocks around it were damaged or burned meant to me that to some people around Kercheval, it was not part of the Establishment. They must then have seen it, at least to some degree, as serving their interests and needs. The Center needed to respond to that expectation now in the confusion of the riot.

But this could not happen if only I wanted it. I spoke to many of the staff by phone Tuesday night, asking them if they would be willing to meet at the Center Wednesday morning. I knew they feared for their safety, but they agreed to come.

I was afraid too, but not for the same reason. I feared that I, so caught up in my own emotions, feeling so wounded by the unbelievable destruction I had seen and smelled and listened to for three days, would not be sensitive to the feelings of the staff toward the rioting and toward me, would not sense the tenor of the neighborhood. I feared that I would say too much or not enough, would do too much or too little, that the Center would not be what it ought to be. As I drove to the Center Wednesday morning, I kept telling myself what I thought I had learned: there was no one way to which everyone would agree as being "best," not my colleagues, nor my friends who were concerned about my safety, nor the staff, nor the various groups in the neighborhood. All I could do was to go and help make the Center ready to respond to whatever unforeseen circumstances might arise.

And to this the staff agreed, although not without misgivings but without my direct urging. Once agreed, they needed little direction outside themselves.

Unlike the year before, professional people did not abandon their clinic services at the Center.

Unlike the year before, black power was being discussed inside and outside the Center. Regardless of whether one advocated violence or nonviolence, black power was no longer a slogan, it was a reality. And a white person could not help but feel that every black person knew it.

When life was in motion at the Center, I left. I went to the central office of the V N A where I could be reached by phone.

I left not for any reasons that I could have given very clearly. It was rather a feeling that Mom and Tots had survived this crisis not because of white people, not because it was sponsored by the Establishment, but because it was black, because it had sought to be responsive to black people. I was an unneeded reminder of the white money and power which black people still needed and resented. But most of all, on that day and increasingly in the days to come, I was not needed.

The white and Negro presses, reflecting varying perspectives, reported the search for causes of what happened, appearing both to agree and disagree. Explanations were sought by labeling the rioting a conspiracy, or variously, as an expression of alienation and frustration, of lawlessness, and of the division among black leaders.

All of the questions directed to me by representatives of a Congressional investigating committee sought reasons for the riot within a conspiratorial framework. When I pointed out this bias to them, they responded by asking whether I was questioning the diligence and earnestness of the committee chairman in Washington. When I assured them that I was not doubting the chairman's intentions to get at the basic causes of the riot, they then asked me what reasons I thought contributed to the riot. Obviously, the kinds of causes which are discovered largely depend on where they are looked for.

A cause-seeking study, completed in Detroit within three weeks after the riot offered reasons beyond conspiracy. The following, based on interviews with 437 Negroes, is a random probability sample of all Negroes fifteen or more years old living in the main riot areas of Detroit. Rioters and nonrioters agreed on the main causes of the riot, out of a list of twenty-three possible grievances. The most frequently chosen were:

(1) police brutality
(2) overcrowded living conditions
(3) poor housing
(4) lack of jobs
(5) poverty
(6) anger with business people

"The conventional liberal idea that rioting is caused by a lack of adequate welfare services was not given very much weight by the majority of Negroes in the survey. Even the riot group ranked this complaint near the bottom (20th)."[6]

The looting which occurred, rather than being regarded simply as lawlessness, has been interpreted as a redefinition of property rights which occurs in three stages.

> Initial looting is often a symbolic act of defiance. The second phase, in which more conscious and deliberate plundering develops, is possibly spurred on by the presence of delinquent gangs that loot more from need or for profit than for ideological reasons. Finally, in the third stage, there is widespread seizure of goods. At this point, looting becomes the socially expected thing to do. . . . The "carnival" spirit observed in the Newark and Detroit disturbances did not represent anarchy. It represented widespread social support for the new definition of property. . . . there is little competition for goods. . . . (it) is quite open and frequently collective. The looters often work together in pairs, as family units, or in small groups.

> At one level, there is no question that looting in civil disturbances is criminal behavior. But the laws that make it so are themselves based on dominant conceptions of property rights. Widespread looting, then, may perhaps be interpreted as a kind of mass protest against our dominant conceptions of property. . . . It is a message that certain deprived sectors of the population want what they consider their fair share—and that they will resort to violence to get it. . . .

> The basic question now is whether American community leaders can or will recognize that such looting is more than "pointless" or "criminal" behavior. . . .[7]

In a basic sense, admittedly abstract and perhaps too self-evident to state, the wide disagreement between and among white and black people over the meaning and causes of urban rioting and consequently what to do about them, is itself symptomatic of the "cause," that is, we do not have a common view of the meaning of human existence and what its quality should be. It means that we look at ourselves and each other as members of our particular race, class, status categories before we view ourselves and others as human beings.

VII
Strengthening the Matrix

"It is necessary while in darkness,
　　to know there is a light somewhere,
　　to know that in oneself,
　　waiting to be found,
　　there is a light"

JAMES BALDWIN

For no man is without strength for expression, and our turning towards him brings about a reply, however imperceptible, however quickly smothered, in a looking and sounding forth of the soul that are perhaps dissipating in mere inwardness and yet do exist.

MARTIN BUBER
from Dialogue

"FOR SALE OR RENT"—Mrs. Vasiloff was trying to get rid of her TV repair shop after the riot. The day-old bakery bricked-in its windows. The cleaners shop protected its new glass with iron gates; so did the grocery and the record shop. The supermarket moved away. The wreckers came and removed the drugstore and the hardware store. The people at Mom and Tots watched the changes, watched Kercheval and McClellan tighten up and brace itself for the future.

The Center was looking different, too. It was extending itself through the wall into the storefront next door, with paint and shelving and play equipment for an enlarged day-care program, and out into the back alley with tar and fencing and climbing toys for a playground, and into the basement with heating and lighting and screening for a recreation room, and into the neighborhood with a new red Volkswagen bus to take families back and forth to downtown clinics.

New doors and floors, new fountain and sink, new wiring, and paint: watermelon and mint, which the children chose, blues and greens, which the women chose; new awnings striped red and white—"You got to get white in there somehow," joked Mrs. Watkins with an almost straight face. And a new sign outside with toy animals designed by Felecia.[1]

New paintings, strung in the window, done by the children, of the riot. Mary Louise overheard two little boys as they walked past the Center: "What's that place?" said one. "Oh," replied the other, "that's an art gallery."

New ties in the neighborhood, to schools and preschools, churches and block clubs, as Mary Louise, now the Center's full-time community worker, made herself acquainted.

New people, coming to the Center—some of them from the food distribution lines.

And new people on the staff.

Mrs. Watkins' neighbor, Sara House, came in the fall. She was the new cook for day care, round and solid, with a twinkle that expressed pleasure when her efforts in the kitchen gave pleasure, as they always did. She didn't know for sure about "protein." But she knew how to pack meals with milk and cheese and eggs without interfering with the flavor of soul food.

And she knew where to find good food at low prices and how to win the battle against roaches. And what did she think about children? Well, a few years back, she found a baby on her doorstep and accepted him as a gift from heaven for her later years.

Mr. Hatt offered to drive the Center's station wagon bus. He was sixty-one, and he had parted with his wife years ago. He lived a few blocks away. Once he'd lived in New York and danced for his living, and could teach with ease, in quiet tones: "You got to try . . . you can dance . . . you can create . . . you ain't never seen a preacher dance like this before. . . ."

He knew the Word, and used it, usually not in vain: "The Book says 'there's a time and a place for everything.' " He knew who he was. "What is your 'first truth'? Your 'first truth' is *you*. My 'first truth' is me, James Hatt." He knew where he came from: "*We* had Soul first—but we're giving some of it to you. . . ." Always in smooth, quiet tones.

Some official people questioned whether Mr. Hatt should be hired. He'd had nine moving violations in five years: five left turns, no brake lights, wrong way on a one-way street, a red light, speeding once. Other official people recalled how they themselves had driven their cars in a similar way, but had been warned or disregarded, rather than ticketed. The staff at Mom and Tots wanted Mr. Hatt. He was hired.

He was on the job—sometimes before 7:30 in the morning when some patients had early appointments at downtown clinics, sometimes after 6 P.M. when patients finished late at clinics—wearing white coveralls, a captain's hat doffed at the right moments, a new set of dentures, and a new pair of eyeglasses.

And Linda came. The day-care staff said, "She's the one." They knew when she walked in the door, Linda MacKay was the one to develop and lead the new ten-hour day-care program. She was twenty-three and very young. Other women had come to apply for the job, mature, poised, experienced women who had raised children of their own. But the staff wanted Linda anyway.

Linda had just finished four years of college in child growth and development. College had been her first experience in a setting that was not all Negro. It was not very comfortable for her.

She loved children. She didn't want to work in the public schools, they were "too structured." She wanted to "make the children proud of themselves. I want to show a child that he can make it on his own, that he can express his feelings freely and openly, and stand up for what he believes, because we Negroes aren't very much able to do this." She pushed back the eyeglasses that had slipped down her nose.

When she saw Mom and Tots, she "felt overjoyed. . . . It's just what I've dreamed of."

She lived at another end of the city. It would take an hour to reach the Center by bus. But it was worth it she said.

Everyone knew that Linda was coming to grow with Mom and Tots.

Mary Louise Moore spread herself over a range of tasks at the Center. She managed to schedule a consistant core of Black obstetricians for the new weekly prenatal clinic, including the president of the International Afro-American Museum Committee (IAM). She no longer questioned the preference of Black over white "outsiders" working at the Center.

She enjoyed instructing Carol Howard in Negro culture: how some middle-income Negro people have kept aloof from the problems of low-income Negro people, how some Blacks had always sought to be "white," straightening their hair, marrying a partner with lighter skin. She once whispered some advice, "When you see us in a group, don't assume we all know each other just because we're Black." It was well taken.

The sons of Pete Collins Jackson came to her. They asked her to visit their mosque with them. She accepted. She'd never been to one before. They asked her where they could find Dan Frank. She told them.

Mary Louise had checked on Dan Frank with Luke and Laine. They thought he was "O.K.," though they didn't know him well.

She visited his ESVID storefront headquarters a few blocks away. Its meeting room was labeled with a big sign

"THINK BLACK!" The walls were covered with reminders as to why and how. Dan said, "You scratch our back, we'll scratch yours." She agreed. He asked her to speak at some block club meetings ESVID was arranging. She did. Referring to her as "Director of Mom and Tots," he described ESVID's prospective program and advised her to "reshape Mom and Tots in order to really bring people in on decisions." At this she blinked her bright black eyes and said, "You seem to be so far ahead of us."

Later, she thought that the Center could probably teach *him* a few things, and besides, he wasn't much of a gentleman since he didn't offer her a chair.

No matter, there was still a lot of common ground for ESVID and Mom and Tots to share.

They both attended the organization session of the City-wide Citizens Action Committee, where "a vision of the new society which Black political rule will initiate" was discussed, and "mass community organizations dedicated to the struggle around immediate grievances . . . (and) . . . the realization of Black political power. . . ."[2] Whites were sifted out at the door. Mary Louise voiced surprise at the number of Black professional people she recognized at the meeting.

Mary Louise calmed Ada Dixon who had heard rumors in the neighborhood that " 'they' (the militants) were going to burn out all the whites that are left."

And Mary Louise tried to raise a question among the staff: "Who am I?"

She had heard the staff talk about Dan Frank: "He talks Black power and Black separation, but he's around whites. . . . What if there *was* a Black state? . . . What about food? Most farmers is white." She heard their feelings and fears about the next generation: how the children need to show initiative, be aggressive, especially the boys, not grow up like the men they know. "And yet," Mary Louise reflected, "they won't tolerate initiative and aggressiveness in their children or their men. . . ."[3]

She was concerned about the sense of identity among Negro people. She considered this a problem for the Center.

Maybe she could work on it with Linda for the sake of the children in day care as well as for their mothers.

She faced other problems and frustrations.

One afternoon she came fuming into the Center. A health agency had denied medications for an unmarried girl who was pregnant and who had asked Mary Louise to help. "They told me 'we're not going to aid and abet these girls to be promiscuous; we won't support whores! After all, *we* work hard for what we have.' " Mary Louise's eyes showed fire as she continued, "And they do it all in the name of God! No wonder the Black Muslims switched to Allah!"

Somehow she always managed to break through agency red tape.

But she had difficulty facing Mr. Hatt. He said, "It ain't so much *what* she say, it's the *way* she say it. She *tells*. . . ." He was a *man* and he wanted to be treated like a man. And it was "mighty hard sometimes, with so many women around." The quietness disappeared from his voice.

And Mary Louise also had a problem facing groups of people, in schools, block clubs, the Center's Mothers Club. "You mean you want me to go *alone?* . . ." "But I've never led a group discussion before. . . ." "Well, I'll try, if you'll be there to give me signals. . . ."

She had another fear: every time Ada Dixon casually, expertly, triumphantly, flicked a roach from the wall to the floor and crunched it with her foot, Mary Louise shivered.

Yet, she laughed about the time someone literally stole the wig off her head as she entered the Center; she could deal with black power with utter finesse; and she could hear between words, the uncertainties of Selfhood trying to express itself.

Energetically, Linda MacKay tackled her new responsibilities, all of them, all at once. She sketched out plans for the new day-care area, walls lined with shelves and bulletin boards, a quiet-corner, a closet for cots and coats. She involved neighborhood women in making new curtains, blankets, aprons for the children.

She enjoyed the children most, and they enjoyed her. They ran to her; they clung to her. She wanted to try to use everything she'd learned in college. She gave them all the feelings she'd held inside for so long.

Sometimes she had to be cautioned not to try to do everything by herself. The other staff members wanted to do their share; her task was to make it possible for them to contribute.

But she complained that the staff wouldn't take responsibility; they left everything to her. And they wouldn't let the children "do for themselves." Mrs. Watkins would never criticize anything, claiming that Linda was "Boss." And why wouldn't Mrs. Watkins take home books to get new ideas? Linda's face showed her distress. She pushed back her glasses —which hadn't slipped—and said, "I just feel like I'm doing something wrong."

She had heard Felecia say, in a strangely aloof manner, "It should be explained (to Linda) that we are not professionals, and the Center cannot be compared to other places. . . ."

Finally, Johnnie West suggested the day-care staff stay one day after the Center closed and meet with Linda privately. Johnnie began, "We aren't reaching our children. We got a special group of children who need lots of loving. But there is something wrong with us, and we got to take care of that first: we're not talking to each other. . . ."

They talked to Linda. "O.K. You want to know what you do wrong: you push too much; you got to relax. . . ." "You got to cool it. . . ." "We start something and you interrupt, 'cause you think you can do it better. . . ."

Linda heard them.

After it was all over, Mrs. Watkins put her arm around Linda, "Now don't take it so hard. . . . And don't worry none about doing somethin' wrong. If you do somethin' wrong, we'll tell you. . . . Next time you got problems, you come to us. You don't need to go upstairs to Whitey. . . . And the reason why I don't want no books is my kids will tear them up and then I got to buy more. . . ."

Almost overnight, there seemed less need for Linda to push back her eyeglasses. She sparkled the Monday morning after

Mrs. Watkins had gone with two of her children to see Linda in a church play.

The staff were busy helping manage the program so they could all spend more time with the children. Johnnie phoned parents. Felecia took attendance. Mrs. Watkins supervised toothbrushing. Mrs. Ford scheduled mothers. Linda collected the fees. "It's not as bad as I thought." Together they interpreted the policies they had set for the all-day program, based on what neighborhood women had suggested, but making exceptions for families in special circumstances. The general rules usually answered most questions:

Reminders for Mothers

1. Obtain a chest x ray.

2. Bring a light blanket and sheet for your child with his name on it.

3. Fees

   WORKING MOTHERS: payment *per day* is equal to the mother's *hourly* pay rate (EXAMPLE: If you make $2 per hour, you will pay $2 per day for your child). Please bring check stub.

   Please pay at the end of each week.

   Please NOTE: If payment is not made after five days, you must talk to the Supervisor, Miss MacKay.

   NONWORKING MOTHERS: You are required to spend at least two hours per week helping in the day-care program. This is in place of paying a fee.

4. Please call if your child is not coming; this will help to plan the meals and the day.

5. Five days of continuous absence without notice

may mean your child will be dropped from enrollment.

Thank you,

Linda MacKay

Mom & Tots Center

But other questions troubled Linda.

Dan Frank's militant ideas frightened her, she couldn't
say how. And Mary Louise had suggested that the children
start talking about the question, "Who am I?" Linda agreed.
But she didn't know how to begin. "I guess I'm not that comfortable about it myself," she said, pushing back her glasses.
She'd talk to the day-care staff.

At first, Felecia laughed at the question, looking at her
arm, "I don't have no trouble about that. . . ." But later she
said that her boy Darrell didn't understand once why she got
so angry when another child called him "nigger," and she
couldn't explain it to him.

Soon even the day-care children were using "Color Me
Brown" books, and looking at picture books with Black children, and posters with Black families. Mary Louise searched
for and found a young Black man, a student teacher, who could
work in the day-care program part time. Linda was happy; Mr.
Hatt was pleased; the staff was glad. But Mrs. Watkins cautioned Linda, "Now don't let him try to run you. . . ."

Linda was pleased they could now discuss racial identity
with the children. She knew that they still needed to tackle the
question of sexual identity. "But how can I talk to the children
about sex," she questioned, "when I can't even talk to the staff
about it?"

A few days before, Mrs. Watkins had laughed quietly as
Linda scanned a new book, *An ABZ of Love*.[4] "Have mercy!"
exclaimed Linda, looking over her glasses, "I'm blushing, but
I got to tell you 'cause you can't tell." All the staff laughed; but
most of them bought a copy of the $7.50 edition.

The staff did seem interested in the topic. Linda thought
perhaps she could approach it by showing them a film on how

parents influence their children's feelings about sex. Maybe the Mothers Club could talk about it, and then they all could be involved in the discussion.

Linda liked the Mothers Club: it helped her organize her thoughts. But she had had trouble accepting her part in it. She was reluctant to lead the group, claiming, "It's not part of my job."

But eventually she recognized that she could not deal with the children in isolation from their parents; she saw that even though she was in charge of the day-care program, it was necessary for her to work with the Mothers Club as well. Each staff member, regardless of his specific job, had to be concerned with the total functioning of the Center: there were no sharp demarcations between their individual areas of responsibility.

Soon Linda was wondering how she could involve the parents more in the day-care program. Perhaps she could have meetings with them once a month, in the evenings. But she worried, "What if they don't come? What if they're not comfortable? What if they don't think their children have gotten anything out of day care?" No, she hadn't really asked the staff for suggestions; she would talk to them.

So the staff met to plan a Parents' Meeting. They decided to help the parents feel welcome and relaxed by using name tags and serving refreshments. The staff could mingle with the group and show the parents the crafts their children were learning. They could discuss the purposes of day care and ask the parents if they had any problems with it.

Linda carried out the staff recommendations. All but two of the parents came. They were enthusiastic: the children were taking better care of toys, sharing more, talking better, eating more foods, watching TV less. They also said their children were less lonely—and that they thought the Center was *theirs*. So did the parents.

Linda beamed.

Late in the fall, Mom and Tots had a new addition to its staff. Mary Louise, with usual graciousness, escorted her around the Center: the new community health nurse, intended to be supervisor, Carlene Williams, B.S., M.P.H.[5] Mary Louise looked out from behind her bright black eyes.

Mrs. Williams was mature, poised, Negro, though not Black. In fact, in her mild Virginia accent, she expressed chagrin that her daughter was about to invite Stokely Carmichael to her wedding. Carlene thought out loud. To her, "black power" was a constructive thing. It meant doing a thing better than a white person did.

She had a pleasant, youthful smile, and laughed, "Looks like I caught hell down there," as the first Negro school nurse in a Southern town twenty-seven years ago. But she thought her best quality was "getting along with all kinds of people." She liked working with people of all ages, and that's what there were at Mom and Tots.

Of course, at her age she had to think about salary, she said. And moving expenses. But she would be willing to take a temporary cut, if the work was something she really wanted to do.

So Mrs. Williams joined Mom and Tots.

In the mornings, she came as early as 7:30, just to chat over coffee with Mrs. Watkins and Mrs. Ford, just to get acquainted; officially she started at 9. But she would leave promptly at 5, because she didn't like to drive all the way across the city in the quickly darkening hours of winter. Mary Louise frequently remained late with children and mothers and often drove Linda home.

After a short time Mrs. Williams had made some observations about the staff: There seemed to be "tension" between Mary Louise and Mr. Hatt; Mrs. Williams thought he was grand with the patients. . . . Linda was not getting all the heights and weights recorded; Mrs. Williams would do them for her. . . . Johnnie was a little late for the prenatal clinics; Mrs. Williams would take care of preparing the examining rooms and charts for the doctor. . . .

Perhaps Mrs. Williams was doing too much for the others. Wouldn't it be better if she encouraged Linda to complete her own records and if she talked to Johnnie about being late? And perhaps there was something she might do to ease the tension between Mary Louise and Mr. Hatt.

Now that Carlene Williams had arrived, Mary Louise and Linda would be able to share the responsibility for leading the Mothers Club sessions with her.

At first Linda had sat in on the Mothers Club sessions as "just part of the group." Then she shared the lead with Mary Louise, who "gave her signals." Now she could say to Mrs. Williams when it was her turn to lead, "Don't worry, it's not so hard. We'll be here to help you."

Together they prepared for the next Mothers Club session.

Linda began. "One problem we have in day care is that parents don't like their boys playing with dolls. Maybe y'all could talk about that. . . ."

The staff considered how they would start out.

"Perhaps we could ask Felecia to role-play," said Mary Louise. "She could dress as a little boy, and play with a doll. Then we could ask the mothers what they would do if that was *their* child. That should get them talking. . . ."

They thought about how the mothers would respond.

"They sure enough wouldn't like it," said Mrs. Williams.

Why?

"They'd be afraid of what would happen to their son," she said.

What would happen?

"He might not grow up normally," she thought.

What does that mean?

"He might be effeminate," Mrs. Williams said.

By "effeminate" do you mean gentle and caring?

"No not just that," she thought. "After all we like our men to be gentle and caring toward us and our children."

Then what are parents afraid of if boys play with dolls?

"Really that he might become perverted," she said.

What does that mean?

"Well, you know, a sissy," Mrs. Williams said.

What does that mean?

"A homosexual," said Mary Louise.

And what is a homosexual?

"Well," thought Mrs. Williams, "someone who has a sexual relationship with a person of the same sex."

And what is not good about that kind of relationship?

"Well, for one thing, for an example," she said, "the people feel guilty and have to be, you know, secretive."

Why do they feel guilty?

"Because society doesn't approve," Linda offered.

Why doesn't society approve?

Linda thought. "You know, I don't know! I guess 'cause it's not natural."

Have you ever loved another girl?

"Sure, you could say so," said Linda. It was her best friend, the only person she could talk to. She never could talk to her mother. But then her friend moved, and she really missed her.

Was that a homosexual relationship?

"Well," Linda thought, "you all could say I liked her, but we never did nothing like that."

Mary Louise said—she had talked about this before— "But you did touch her, maybe you hugged or kissed her when she left?"

"Sure, when she left. I told you I really missed her," Linda said.

"So in a way, that was a homosexual relationship, though it certainly wasn't 'perverted' whatever that means," Mary Louise said cautiously.

How many kinds of relationships can anyone have?

"I suppose, when you come down to it," Mary Louise thought out loud, "you can only relate to people of the opposite sex or to people of the same sex—so there are either heterosexual or homosexual kinds of relationships."

Can heterosexual relationships be bad?

"Can they!" said Mrs. Williams. "I guess a man and a woman can be as mean to each other as a man to a man or a woman to a woman."

"Or they sure can be good for each other too," said Linda.

Linda, did you ever feel close to a man?

"Ya," she said slowly, "I just met somebody two weeks ago. But we aren't doing anything. . . ."

Does he know how you feel?

"Ya. . . ."

How does he know?

"Oh, I just talk and talk to him, and he talks to me, and we just do more and more things together. And I know he really cares about me 'cause he say he'll wait 'til I'm ready."

But you do feel close to each other now?

"Oh, ya. . . ."

"In other words," Mrs. Williams said, "people can be intimate with each other without being physically intimate."

"Or they can be physically intimate without really knowing each other at all, no matter what their sexes," thought Mary Louise.

"Well, then," Mrs. Williams questioned, "what is the right thing? What *are* we going to tell the mothers?"

Is there a right thing to tell them? Or shall we just let them see that there are alternative ways of looking at behavior?[6]

Linda thought that they should have the chance to decide for themselves, even though that gets confusing sometimes.

As staff meeting started, Ada Dixon looked at Felecia, "What y'all lookin' evil about? It's Christmas, Baby!"

"Well," said Felecia, "I'm not happy. You know when we took the day-care children to see Santa last week at Hudson's Toyland? Well, yesterday when the Center had its party for the neighborhood, little Kim said to me after she got her present from our Santa, 'That's not the real Santa 'cause he doesn't have a white face.' "

Mary Louise looked out of her bright eyes, "Perhaps Mr. J. L. Hudson, Jr. ought to be made aware that some Santas ought to have black skin. Maybe we ought to send him a letter suggesting that for next Christmas."

The staff agreed. . . .

Johnnie said, "Tommie Sanderson thought all our new

renovations were 'pretty.' He wanted to do something too. So I let him paint the file cabinet. I think that was all right."

The staff agreed. . . .

"I got something to say," said Ada. "Mrs. Jefferson and I was thinking that them kids need something more in that recreation room in the basement. We was just wondering if maybe you all thought the Center could afford to get maybe a ping-pong table. I know where there's one, cheap."

The staff agreed. . . .

Linda said, "I want to know what y'all think of Mrs. Peters in day care yesterday. I don't think she's right for the children. Look at the way she dresses. . . ."

Mrs. Peters was a new addition to the staff, a mother of four who lived not far away. She wore a narrow-brimmed hat, always tilted to one side, and sometimes high, snug boots with short skirts, or neatly fitted pant-suits. She came as a substitute for the clinic sessions and for day care.

"I don't want to take sides. . . . Oh, I'd better not say, . . ." Felecia hesitated.

"Go on, Felecia," urged Mrs. Watkins quietly.

"Well, everyone have different personalities," Felecia went on, "and it took all of us time to get used to the children when we first started, so we should give her a chance too. . . ."

And they did.

The
Center
was

resurgent. You could feel it. It
was not just the feeling of relief from having survived crises in
breathless succession. It was a sense of new life, of freshness; a
readiness to start again and be better than we were before. The
staff members were more consistently sharing their strengths with
each other; Johnnie's maturity and intelligence, Felecia's suc-
cinctness, the strength of Mrs. Watkins' mothering, Mr. Hatt's
charm and attentiveness—each expressing in his own way that
nameless something, the legacy of blackness, called "soul."[7] They
were no longer hesitant to express their pride in its source.

As they took hold, I receded. After the riot, I spent about
four or five hours a day at the Center. I could always be reached
by phone, but in time, the phone calls diminished to almost none.
In planning the new Center, how it should look and feel, Mary
Louise worked with neighborhood groups. I had long since relin-
quished direct contact with patients in the clinics or children in
the clubs. In hiring new people, I awaited the recommendations
by the staff of persons they knew or of those who periodically
stopped in to ask for a job. In supervising the staff, I now worked

primarily through Mary Louise, Linda, and Carlene Williams.

I could also indirectly infuse questions and ideas into the Center which at an earlier time and in a more direct fashion were too threatening, such as making the meaning of blackness explicit, dealing with sexuality openly, finding ways to involve parents, patients, children, and each other in decision-making. I did this principally in two ways: through individual conferences and through the Mothers Club sessions.

I had individual meetings with Mary Louise, Linda, and Mrs. Williams at least once a week, where I could give my complete attention to their concerns. Our conversations lasted one to two hours, and I almost never allowed myself or them to let other goings on take priority. I tried to focus on the interpersonal problems they presented, not the "mechanical" ones; not what should they buy in a particular circumstance, but how would they go about deciding what they should buy; not the listing of petty complaints, but what were the bases for the difficulties, in themselves, in others, in the situation, and how they could proceed to change these. My dilemma was always how far I should allow their difficulties to progress in order to provide the impetus for them to seek their own resolution. It was difficult to know how long I should wait before intervening with a suggestion or a decision. In time, the need for my suggestions diminished.

Mary Louise began to learn to talk directly. After many months, I could ask her whether she was aware that she often spoke in the passive voice grammatically, and used pronouns rather than nouns, making her speech sound removed and vague. She began to observe this in herself, and its implications, and to point this out about herself to me. She began to speak more directly about black people and black power. For whatever reasons, she lost her naiveté and became increasingly knowledgeable about black politics in Detroit. She and Linda became the ones to make explicit the question "Who am I?" for the older staff members, and then through the Center's programs. I watched her make step-by-step progress with this, as she also painfully faced her fear of talking in front of a group. We took that in steps, too: she first watched me, then led a group with me, then I watched her, then she was on her own and would later describe the meetings to me.

Way in the beginning, when Mary Louise first came to the Center, we both, but she more than I, had to shed the horseblinders worn by many professional people: the notion that if you are in one category you cannot perform the functions of another. She was originally a licensed practical nurse, and thus thought she was not capable of doing what registered nurses usually do, such as lead a group discussion on health, or give a baby bath demonstration. Without the hindrance of labels and uniforms, Mary Louise functioned ably. She became my colleague, one whose perceptions and evaluations I listened to.

The first few months of my sessions with Linda were painful for both of us. She probably had not had much opportunity to talk at length before, nor to be listened to. She was alternately eager and enthusiastic, angry and sullen, and always raw, like the growing edge of a wound, jagged, tender, but alive. After the meeting at which the day-care staff confronted her, which she and others described to me later, Linda began to unfold. It was not a smooth development, but it was visible, I and others could see it; and most importantly, Linda knew it.

She could become angry with me directly, and she could also examine why she was angry. She talked openly and was open to new ideas. She raised thoughtful questions and was willing to think about the questions I raised with her. Her difficulties with the meaning of authority—of relating to authority-figures, as well as being in a position of supervising others—were obvious enough; but she was willing eventually to talk openly with the staff about this and let them help her.

Linda's wish for absolute lines of responsibility, for rigid divisions, is as impossible of fulfillment in an organization where people are working together toward wholeness as it is in society. There is an eternal interdependence, a complex complementarity, which must produce dis-ease when it is denied.

Carlene Williams was among the best of her generation, dedicated to her work, persistent, tenacious, determined to "make it." She had "made it," she had more than once quietly worked toward attainment in the white world, swallowing her anger and resentment. But, consistent with her way of doing, she was also nonassuming, not directly aggressive, and consequently had her own problems about authority. It was many months before she could admit to some of her anger. But she was willing to talk and to hear questions which in her own mind had been settled and set aside. I hoped she could share herself with the others and draw support from them; I hoped she could take off the horse-blinders of professionalism.

The Mothers Club sessions provided another opportunity to foster a quality of life in the people and programs at the Center. The pattern which had emerged involved a preparatory discussion among the staff who were to lead the group; the group session itself which consisted of neighborhood women and the Center's core staff; and immediately afterward, an evaluation of the dynamics by the group leaders. The leaders were usually paired, one was primarily responsible for the discussion material and for maintaining the flow of the session, the other was to listen, give cues, and help evaluate.

Mary Louise, Linda, and Mrs. Williams as alternating leaders met together with me in the preparatory discussions. The discussion topic was chosen by the previous Mothers Club session. I think we all enjoyed these discussions; they were lively and re-laxed. I could raise questions that they had perhaps not thought about, and they could think their new thoughts out loud. My aim continued to be to provide a broader range of possibilities for them, and through them for the mothers and the other staff people, and through them for the other programs, the clinic groups, day care, the clubs. The reminder was always given, to allow people out of the scope of the possible to choose their own best way.

I was not a part of the Mothers Club sessions, but I could listen from my desk in the corner.

The four of us afterward had a twenty to thirty-minute evaluation in terms of the reactions to the ideas that had been discussed, the perceptions of others' reactions, and the skill of the group leader in directing but not dominating the discussion. These meetings were uniquely free of defensiveness and criticism. They seemed very pleased with the development of their own leader-ship abilities and were ready to define where they could improve the next time. Some of the Center's healthiest glow showed through the pattern and process of those group sessions.

As a result of the discussions before the various kinds of groups at the Center, ideas once avoided became normal and natural in the ordinary flow of conversation; whether of black and white, male and female, dominance and submission, self and other, loving and hating; and most importantly, the variations and complexities between and among these.

VIII
Wholeness Unfolding

Joy is the emotional expression of the courageous
Yes to one's own true being.

PAUL TILLICH
from *The Courage To Be*

Like the expert she was, Mrs. House flipped the tiny pancakes she was preparing for the children's morning snack in day care. She was proud of her kitchen and kept it sparkling. Now it was separated from the play area by a partition of translucent blue and green plastic squares that could be raised and lowered over the counter.

The children came up to the ledge and helped themselves to their snack. They had just come in from a fire drill, a little routine that Mary Louise and Linda added to the program. This afternoon they were going to the Civic Center to see the Mobile Museum of the International Afro-American Museum Committee. Mary Louise was now a member of I A M.

Next week Linda was planning to use the slides on *How Babies Are Made*. The children in day care would learn about reproduction in chickens, dogs, and people from the slides. Then they would go to a farm. It would be a new experience for the staff and most of the parents, as well as for the children. Everyone was looking forward to it, especially Linda.

As soon as the pancakes were finished, and while the children were trying out the Mexican Hat Dance, Mrs. House began lunch: cream of celery soup, baked chicken, sweet potatoes, cabbage, milk, and applesauce.

Ada had sneaked down to day care and with a wink to Mrs. House grabbed a paper plate of pancakes. As she tiptoed back upstairs, Mrs. Williams saw her, and the two of them shared the snack.

Mary Louise, busy on the phone, looked longingly at the dish. As usual, she knew she'd feel guilty if she interrupted her perpetual reducing diet.

Little Tommie Sanderson stopped upstairs at lunchtime to empty the wastebaskets. Mrs. Williams noticed the back of his head. "Tommie, how long has your head been like that? Doesn't it hurt?"

He didn't know how long, but it sure did pain him.

It looked to her like a fungus with a secondary bacterial infection.

"Mary Louise, let's see what we can do for Tommie," she said.

Several phone calls and notes later, neither had been able to reach Mrs. Sanderson. No one at the Center had ever seen her. She hadn't been home when Mary Louise stopped at the house.

"What do you think we should do now?" Mrs. Williams wondered.

Together they made an appointment for Tommie for the next day at a PRESCAD pediatric clinic, arranged for Mr. Hatt to pick him up at his house, explained it all to Tommie who was eager to get rid of the pain, and sent a note to his mother asking her to be ready to go with him.

After the examination at the clinic, a smiling Mrs. Sanderson brought Tommie back to the Center to show Mrs. Williams and Mary Louise the medicine the doctor had prescribed for his infected scalp.

At the Cleaners down the street, Ada overheard a woman say how worried she was because she didn't have enough money to buy medicine; her family doctor hadn't asked her about that, when he prescribed it for her sick child. Ada brought the mother back to Mom and Tots. She asked Mr. Hatt to take the lady downtown to City health services where there would be no charge for the medicine.

The child had his medicine within two hours.

The mother was grateful. She was going to tell all her neighbors about Mom and Tots.

The Nichols Elementary School PTA wanted to hear more about Mom and Tots. Mary Louise and Linda and Johnnie spent an evening telling them.

The Pingree School Pre-Teen Girls wanted to know what Mom and Tots could teach about sexuality. Mary Louise led a discussion with them and their mothers, sixty-five altogether. They wanted her to come back. She would be happy to, but she inquired with her usual diplomacy whether they would like her to bring a young Black man with her, perhaps a medical student. Then the girls could get more realistic answers to their questions on sexuality.

The Michigan Welfare League in the state capitol wanted

to know about Mom and Tots. Would Mrs. Watkins like to talk to them? "Well, I'd have to pray about it first," she said.

The next day she said, "Well, I do like to ride, and I ain't never been to Lansing. . . ."

She went. She talked to about seventy-five health and welfare professionals and lay people, with just a little quiver in her voice.

She was pleased. On the drive back to Detroit she said, "I guess the words was just given to me." She chattered on and on about how hard things were for so long, about how much better things were now that her husband needed only to work one job. With a straight face she said, "It ain't so bad bein' poor, it's just so darn inconvenient."

The O E O Family Planning Division in Chicago wanted to hear about Mom and Tots. Would Johnnie like to go? Her eyes brightened; then, she hesitated. She'd have to think about it.

The next day, she said, "I don't know how I can tell you so you'll understand . . . it would be a wonderful thing . . . but it's different when you're married. . . . My husband won't let me go. . . . He's jealous. . . ."

The City Health Department came to ask Mom and Tots for help. Could they use the Center for an evening immunization clinic once a month? Of course, they could.

Johnnie thought the whole thing was "beautiful." She talked to the mothers about the Center's prenatal and family planning services as the women waited in line with their children. The Teen Club helped babysit. Mrs. Williams helped swab the arms. Linda offered toys to amuse the youngsters. And Mary Louise cuddled them after they'd received their shots. Then there was Tommie Sanderson, directing traffic—189 people had come in two hours, including his mother with four of her children.

ESVID had agreed to tell its members about Mom and Tots' immunization clinic, though not about the birth-control services. But recently, Mary Louise had been working with

ESVID's new welfare organizer, a woman who was also chairman of the Committee on Humanizing Existing Assistance Rules (HEAR), and a mother of six. She was more sympathetic to family planning than Dan Frank was.

Bernard, Felecia's husband, had volunteered to sponsor the Boys' Club on Saturdays, when he wasn't working. Regi had been drafted into the army. Mary Louise was pleased to see that Bernard had let the boys elect officers. She had talked to him about how important it was for them to make their own decisions, help plan their activities, and spend their five-dollar-a-month budget. She also stressed how they should have a chance to say what they felt about being Black; and how he should answer all their questions straight, even sex questions. Bernard, tall and handsome and self-confident, was the man to do it. In their recreation room, with the new ping-pong table, was a big picture of Cassius Clay. The boys talked about what they hated, and also about what made them happy.

Laine Thomas had left Mom and Tots for a full-time job of teaching and then marriage. She had recommended a friend to take her place. This young woman left for college after a few months. Mary Louise found another leader for the teens—Ann Jones.

Ann hadn't "gone natural," as Laine and her friend had. In fact, Ann didn't know what "Afro-American" meant. She had been suggested to Mary Louise by the wife of a minister from a nearby Baptist church. But Ann was interested and wanted to work with the teens. Mary Louise would work with her.

Within six weeks Ann was talking to the girls about what they thought was most important in their lives. She asked them to write down their thoughts. These were her own:

> To me love is first on the list of important things in my life. Next is people, and without the help of others I couldn't survive alone in this world. . . .

There are so many things I am not fully aware of and not familiar with. I feel that when you've been brought up in a somewhat limited life with few activities, it's hard to get away; especially when the parents don't participate in different activities and don't encourage their children to do so. This means that the child would have to learn about different activities from others, which doesn't guarantee that the parents will understand. . . .

Another thing which I feel is of vital importance to me is respect. If you can't respect yourself you cannot respect others or expect others to respect you.

Another thing that is important to me is happiness, things you like to see and do, and sentiments that are derived from the things you do and see, make you happy. And to be happy is a good feeling.

I am also proud of what I am, a Negro in the middle class of society. The Negro race is one of the most colorful and beautiful races of this day. We are not just one color but a mixture of many.

Ann began to think about the meaning of "black power" as she talked with Mary Louise. It no longer had such a terrifying ring, it no longer meant violence.

After six months Mrs. Williams commented, "Ann really talks their language" as she saw Ann lead the teens in a discussion. Of the dozen teenagers who met, the boys outnumbered the girls. Ann could allow them to express ideas which were sometimes distinctly contrary to her own. . . .

A boy, 17: I think sex is fine. Naturally teenagers is going to have sex relations. I don't see nothing wrong with it. Now when a boy meets a girl, after he has known her for a little while, you know, been talking to her, he's going to run her down the line. . . .

A girl, 16: I feel the same way. Nothing is wrong with having sex but you should know how to protect yourself from getting pregnant. Or the boy should protect you. . . .

Ann: What do you mean by "protecting" yourself?

A girl, 16: I mean the girl, she ought to see that the boy uses a rubber. Or some girls take pills or go to the drugstore and get something.

Ann: Are you saying that every boy friend you have, it is all right to have a sexual relationship?

A girl, 16: I don't think you should have a sexual relationship with every boy friend, but when you are older and going steady and plan to get married then it's all right. Because there is responsibility in getting married and most time when a girl get pregnant she and her mother has to take care of the baby. Sometimes you don't even know where the boy is. . . .

A boy, 17: Well I don't plan to get married but I agree that the boy he should help to take care of the baby. That's another reason why girls should not have sex unless they know what they're doing. Girls should talk with their mothers about such things. . . .

A girl, 16: Oh no! You can't discuss or talk with your mother because the first thing they think is you are pregnant. . . .

A girl, 17: That's right. I don't see why mothers always feels you is going to get pregnant. They was young once. . . .

Ann: In other words, what you all are saying is that you don't feel like anything is wrong with sex if you are going steady and plan to marry. You admit it is hard to talk with your mothers. But mothers is more understanding than you sometimes think. Also, fathers can give you a lot of advice. . . .

A boy, 13: Yes, last night I wanted to talk to my Daddy because a man was parked in a car and called me but I didn't go. Then he told another boy to tell me he would give me a dollar if I would suck him. I got scared and ran.

A boy, 14: Ya, man, I know what you all mean. A man

asked me to do the same thing but I told him he was crazy. . . .

A girl, 16: One boy at school told me a male teacher offered him ten dollars if he would go to bed with him. . . . And another thing, you hear a lot of talk now about boys and girls using their mouths on your privates. To me that is nasty. . . .

Mrs. Williams met with the teens once a month. She was willing to bend to help bridge the generational gap, to "talk their language."

Mrs. Williams planned the weekly prenatal clinic sessions with Johnnie and Mary Louise, and a practical nurse from the V N A district office, whose only fault was that she thought she had to talk in order to teach—but the Center was showing her otherwise. Sometimes the obstetricians would want to join the discussion. One of them said quietly to Mrs. Williams that he was glad there was a Negro supervisor at Mom and Tots.

Johnnie had put up new bulletin boards. She wanted them to say important things, but things that made the ladies comfortable. In the examining rooms she had:

Our doctor is your friend:
>Talk to him
>Ask him questions
>Relax

and pictures of Black children which she labeled "Your Child's Rights."

In the reception area were signs saying "Have a Normal Baby by Keeping Healthy" and "Keep Your Family Healthy."

One Wednesday morning in early spring, 1968, Ada realized by 9:30 that Mrs. Williams would probably not be coming in; she had been out of the city for a funeral. This was prenatal clinic day, so she called Mrs. Peters to come and help set up the clinic. Mrs. Peters came, smartly attired as always.

Everything was ready by 10, when the patients came, and the patients were ready for the obstetrician when he came at 10:30.

Late in the day, Mrs. Williams came in. How did things

go? Mrs. Peters described how she'd enjoyed helping the ladies. This was her first time as "clinic assistant" under Johnnie's direction.[1] Johnnie told how she had decided to include in her discussion with the ladies a detailed description of the two Black hospitals that were now providing Mom and Tots with delivery services. "I tell them I'm glad for the opportunity to work with our own color," she said. They were all pleased.

But there was one problem, Ada added. The bathroom faucet was still leaking. She tapped the screwdriver in her hand, "I been screwing all day," she grinned and rolled her eyes.

Mrs. Williams gave a full chuckle, "Then you must be feeling mighty good by now—and you're still on your feet!"

It was one of Mary Louise's jobs to make necessary contacts with the landlady,[2] and the next morning she had Mrs. Vasiloff's son upstairs about the faucet. "No," Mary Louise insisted, "it's your responsibility. . . . Our lease says. . . ."

He repaired it.

There were now three birth-control clinic sessions each week.[3] Johnnie would talk to the women while the Planned Parenthood doctor and nurses worked in the examining rooms. Old Mrs. McGovern had gone, and in her place was a young blond nurse who thought Mom and Tots was "great." She and Johnnie learned from each other.

Johnnie showed Mrs. Peters how she worked with the groups of women during the family-planning clinics. Sometimes the discussions centered on the care of young children, sometimes on sexual problems with their husbands. One woman told Johnnie, "I ain't been able to have relation with my husband for awhile. . . . I wouldn't be able to talk about it once, but this has helped me a lot. . . ."

Sometimes Johnnie talked with them about the rights of children, and of women:

> . . . a child should have I would say six rights or seven. . . .
> Number one is food, they need the right kind of food to grow
> and be healthy. . . . Number two will be health care, which
> they should see a doctor ever so often. . . . Number three
> would be a home, and a nice home, a place to grow and live

in. . . . Number four would be education, and other than high-school education, even if they want to go to college. . . . Number five would be moral and spiritual guidance, because so many families relies on school or churches or something. We need this at home to teach the child how to be and how to live. . . . Number six would be clothing because children grow and they tear clothes and it is expensive. . . . Number seven is love, and included with love is time to give each child a little of you, a little closeness, just make that child feel extra special. . . .

And you have your own rights; because if you have a house-ful of children you don't have time for yourself, you don't have time for your husband, and just about all your time is taking care of a family and cleaning up and cooking and that's the way the day ends and the day begins, nothing really to look forward to and nothing to look back on. . . .

One of the requests that had come from the day-care parents was for more discussion on discipline. So Linda led one of the spring Mothers Club meetings on "How Do You Punish Your Child?" Twenty-five women, including some of the Mom and Tots staff, sat snugly around the reception area upstairs.

"The way we discipline our children is the way they'll discipline themselves," she began. "If we're rigid, they'll be like this," she stiffened her body. "We as Negroes are rigid," she continued, "but we need to find our *own* way of doing things . . . we need to be free . . . creative; there's not just one right way that someone else tells us. This is the way we need to raise our children."

"I think we can be too hard on our children," said Johnnie. "As parents we say 'No' and we really want the child to accept 'No.' If he is raised as the kind of child who is used to accepting 'No,' he is not going to try to fight for what he wants; he is just going to take 'No.' But when we say 'No' I feel we should at least give the child a chance to explain himself, why the answer should be 'Yes'. . . ."

". . . Most of us don't go within ourselves and ask ourselves 'why?' (do we want a child to do a thing)," another mother said.

One mother described how she'd heard her little boy say "bull shit," which he'd heard her say. So she washed out both their mouths with soap.

They continued for almost two hours.

As the discussion ended, a mother of five said, "When I come here I thought I had a problem, but now that I heard *you* all, I don't have no problems."

In the staff meeting at the end of the week, Felecia said, "I don't mean to show no favors or nothing, but Tommie Sanderson's birthday is coming, and I thought maybe we could have a little party for him, just a little one, because really, he's done so much for us. . . . What you all think?"

"And he doesn't get angry no more like he used to when we ask him to leave," Linda added.

"Truly," said Ada.

"That's sure enough," said Mrs. Watkins.

"And I can make homemade ice cream," offered Mrs. House.

Mary Louise's eyes glowed softly.

Mrs. Williams smiled brightly.

Sometimes it was difficult to disagree.

The Center was

more than pleasant to be in. For me, in the last months that I was there, it was brightness and warmth, openness and freedom, a place where people could be themselves. It seemed alive to me. I think it was what many of the people around it wanted it to be, which is one of the reasons it was what I wanted it to be.

I enjoyed going there in the mornings. One morning, just a few weeks before I was to officially end my relationship with the Center, I stopped in the day care area, as I always did before going upstairs. As usual, I went to the kitchen counter in the back where I greeted Mrs. House, with a good word for the delicious smells coming from her pots and pans. As always she smiled broadly and offered me my favorite kind of homemade cooky: the crispiest remains from yesterday, meaning the burnt crumbs. But she had saved a very large "crumb" for me that morning.

As usual, I walked over to say good morning to the staff, asking Mrs. Watkins how Deneen was doing in pre-school now, complimenting Mrs. Ford on her attractive hair.

All of a sudden, eight or ten little children who had been

playing elsewhere surrounded me, all shouting "I want some!" "Me too!" pointing to the cookie in my hand. Even though I held it high, they could almost reach it since I am not much taller than some of them. They were gentle in their tumbling about, on and over the blocks and toys.

"We can all have some if everyone takes just a little piece," I said.

So I squatted and held the burnt molasses cookie as each child took a tiny piece. The last piece was mine. We munched the crisp bits together. Then they all ran back to play.

I was caught up in my thoughts.

I never spoke of that little incident. It was hardly noticeable. It would have seemed mildly ludicrous to many people to attach any significance to it.

Nevertheless, and in spite of my having severed any ties with the church a long time ago, somewhere in that incident was a kind of communion which helped me prepare finally to leave the Center.

IX
Transition

The moment we cease to hold each other,
the moment we break faith with one another,
the sea engulfs us and the light goes out.

JAMES BALDWIN

For the Center, to unfold meant to change, not only in its dynamics and structure, but in its status as a "project." For the Mom and Tots Center to move from "project" to ongoing organization meant, among other things, replacing the project director with a supervisor.

Two years after the Center started, the transition began to be discussed, with Mary Louise, with Linda, with Ada, with Mrs. Williams, and then with the staff as a whole.

"I'm shocked! . . ."

"So am I. . . ."

One turned away, almost in tears.

Linda straightened herself, "Now look here, you all. This is black power isn't it—if we can't go on alone, then we really didn't do it. . . ."

"But it isn't like she's White. . . ."

"We gonna be here and we gonna carry right on. . . ." Ada stood up to talk.

Mary Louise was silent. She slowly wrote a note to herself "How to act without Nancy in the building."

As she went out, Mrs. Watkins said, "All I got to say is 'God bless you,' Girl."

In the weeks and months that followed came their reactions to Mrs. Williams as their prospective supervisor. The change would be official on April 1, 1968.

I just feel like things is changing and I don't like the feeling nohow. . . .

She think she going to be boss over the whole Center. . . .

I only got one boss. . . .

These colored people with "education". . . .

What happens if we don't agree with her? . . .

Mary Louise reacted:

I don't feel anything . . . so I can't say how I feel. . . .

Sometimes I'd like to say to her 'O.K., if you want to be boss then you do *all* the thinking'. . . .

185

It's frustrating to have to try to express my feelings in front of her. . . .

And then Mary Louise's back began to bother her. It used to hurt when she worked at the V N A District Office. She stayed home a couple of days, a rare occurrence. She went to the doctor. She might have to be hospitalized to find out what was wrong.

Mary Louise was reminded that Mrs. Williams had been willing to move to Detroit to work at Mom and Tots, with a cut in pay. . . . Were there *specific* things Mary Louise was afraid of?

Mrs. Williams reacted to the others. Sometimes she'd laugh buoyantly, "I'm being tried and tested." Sometimes she was downcast:

I don't feel I'm a part of the Center. . . .

I want the respect everyone else has. . . .

I want to be known as supervisor; after all this is my specialty; this is what I was educated for . . . all my classmates have supervisory positions. . . .

Mary Louise is so sullen . . . she's charming to visitors, but not to us. . . . I think that's dishonest. . . . I feel smothered when she plops her materials on my desk. . . . What will we do if she goes into the hospital? . . .

And then her stomach began to bother her; she knew it hurt whenever she encountered a new situation. She stayed home more than a few days. She went to the doctor. The medicine helped.

Ada Dixon was looking distressed. She wanted to talk, alone. She was upset by the tension between Mrs. Williams and Mary Louise. Who was "higher"? She wanted to know. Yes, she knew it would take time and that everyone had their strengths and weaknesses. She remembered the beginning of the Center. Well, she was glad she was able to say it anyway, instead of "stewing and fretting."

Mrs. Williams came back to the Center.

Did she think she was helping Ada by expressing her frustrations to her? . . . Perhaps she could help Mary Louise by supporting the person she *wants* to be. . . . How could she help the staff organize themselves if Mary Louise should go into the hospital?

"We all got to know how things are going to be decided around here," Linda stated.

She was right. How *were* things going to be decided? Would she want to appeal to the director of the VNA if she couldn't resolve an issue with Mrs. Williams?

Linda thought she would call a meeting of the staff to discuss it.

Mary Louise said she knew she'd have to be speaking more with Mrs. Williams. She suggested to Mrs. Williams that the two of them meet together once a week. They did. At first politely. Then, Mary Louise spoke out, "You don't need to be angry like the rest of us, you've got everything. . . ."

"Now let me tell you," said Mrs. Williams, "everything I have I worked for and fought for. . . ."

In later talks Mrs. Williams asked, "What are you going to do about these vague fears? . . ." And, "I'm here to stay, and I won't be going until I'm ready to go. . . ." Or, "You did beautifully leading that discussion on 'Who Am I?' with the Mothers Club. . . ."

Sometimes the staff would bolster Mrs. Williams. "You know how our people are," Mrs. House told her, "just be firm. . . . It's just like in church, some people wants to take it all over. . . ." Or Mr. Hatt would softly tell her, "You know how to treat a man like a man. . . ."

Mary Louise invited Mrs. Williams to a sorority meeting to hear Julian Bond, the Black legislator from Georgia. As they descended the steep staircase leading away from the hotel luncheon meeting, Mrs. Williams took Mary Louise's arm for fear of falling. "Looks like if we go down, we go down together," she said. They turned and looked straight at each other.

In staff meeting Mrs. Williams made clear that she, too, wanted to be called by her first name. And she confessed she had been wearing her community health nursing uniforms only because she thought she "was supposed to" during clinics; but now she was going to "throw those drab old things out" and wear the bright clothes she wanted to wear.

Linda told Mrs. Williams that everyone had discussed what would happen if they disagreed on a certain issue.

"I thought we should cross that bridge when we come to it," said Felecia.

But Johnnie had thought they should try to look further ahead than that and foresee what would be done.

Mary Louise had felt that even if well-intentioned, an outsider (like the VNA director) wouldn't quite know enough to help resolve a disagreement.

Mrs. Watkins summed it up, "In other words, we're gonna solve all our problems right here. We'll just fight it out among ourselves if we got to. We don't need no outsider telling us how to do. . . ."

Carlene Williams was satisfied.

Felecia added, "Don't worry, everyone feel pretty good about you."

April 1 passed without event.

Individually and as a group the staff attended to the problems and possibilities connected with the change.

Then on April 4 Martin Luther King was killed.

The next day Linda forced herself to go to the Center. She knew the children would need her. She knew she'd have to explain, so it would make sense, something that did not make sense.

Trying to contain her own feelings, she gathered the children around her. How did they feel when their Mommy or Daddy or brothers or sisters went away? . . .

Had they seen the TV? . . .

Everyone was going to be very sad, she told them. But because of Martin Luther King "you all can grow up with a feeling of being great."

Linda had brought a poem with her. It was written during the night by an unknown young man, a friend of a friend. She read it to the children:

> A man's been killed in Tennessee
> He gave his life so we'd be free. . . .
> Whose work on earth will never cease
> Until this nation unites in peace.
>
> He marched, he talked to spread the word
> At times ridiculed and considered absurd. . . .
>
> He loved his people, he loved his God
> He loved this earth on which he trod
> He tried to equalize his race
> To make this world a better place. . . .

At noon the Mom and Tots staff gathered upstairs quietly for staff meeting. Johnnie was worried. Rioting was going on in Memphis. Memphis was home to her.

Ada suggested that the Center close for the funeral next Tuesday. Everyone agreed.

Mrs. Williams asked each person what she felt. She tried to put into words the sense of loss.

Linda wanted to read the poem. Everyone listened quietly. She got half-way through it:

> Who, in this earthly place we live,
> Would take such a life God chose to give?
> For such a man to leave this earth
> Makes you wonder how much it's worth. . . .

and she cried. She couldn't read anymore.

Sitting near her, Mrs. Watkins reached over and took the

poem from Linda. She continued to read for Linda, quietly, smoothly, clearly:

> Don't cry for King, he knew no fear
> Weep for this world that we live in here.
>
> The world has lost a gracious man
> Who helped his people throughout the land;
> All he wanted was equality;
> Keep in mind, he died for you and me.

It
is
dangerous

to encourage people to talk—to express their feelings in words, to shape their ideas into coherent forms. The person in charge cannot predict what will happen; he cannot control the words. It is an open situation, and everyone becomes more vulnerable, more exposed, and thus more equal.

And the whole process is threatening to people. They will be frightened by their own feelings, by their fears and longings, and by the possibilities of their own ideas. Hearing themselves talk raises new expectations of themselves and their circumstances. They will no longer be satisfied with being given answers and being told what to do. And once they have begun, they will expect to continue to talk and to criticize.

It is threatening to the person in charge. He cannot stay the same. Nothing is ever over and done with, final, completed. He must continue responding to a changing milieu: sometimes the change is erratic, sometimes it is flowing, but always there is movement. As he hears people learning to talk with their souls, he has an awesome responsibility: he must listen and help them focus and channel what comes before them both. It cannot remain in limbo. For this he needs his best energies, his most alert self. They will expect it. As he hears the hopes and anxieties of others, the leader in charge will recognize the similarities with his own situation; and then he has his own self to deal with.

The whole process is inherently dangerous. Only a belief in the human rightness of it, in its importance to human wholeness, makes it worth the effort.

Having developed an expectation for talking-listening at the Center, I wanted to provide the means for it to continue consciously after I was gone. After discussion with the staff, a mental health consultant, a young white woman, was invited to come regularly to the Center. Apart from her professional credentials as a graduate instructor in child psychiatric nursing, the consultant was qualified, to my mind, because she accepted the philosophy of the Center as well as her status as an outsider; she had had experience working in a ghetto, and most importantly, she was the only visitor to the Center to receive the explicit, unsolicited approval of the staff. As Felecia said, referring to her, "Everyone don't *have* to be black."

The staff saw her as coming primarily to help them understand the interactions of the children in day care. My hope was that this would allow them the opportunity to continue to look at themselves and their relationships with each other, as well as help ease the inevitable discomforts of the transition phase.

Other structural arrangements which I made in preparation for my leaving were centralizing certain mechanical procedures, as I have described (see p. 206), and dissolving the position of project director. This in effect required the VNA to assume more of the time-consuming paper work, as well as the worries of adequate funding. The VNA could no longer view the Center as a tentative "project" but as an established entity which expressed the VNA's concern for health. The VNA would carry the responsibility for its financial and structural support. The new person in charge of the Center needed to be a supervisor—one who was responsible for the quality of relationships and development of people. She should not have to be encumbered with administrative problems as well. By using the term "supervisor" I hoped to minimize for Carlene Williams the difficulty of being viewed as "replacing" me, either in function or personality. The Center no longer required either the personality or functions of a "project director."

After April 1, I no longer went to the Center. To aid in the transition, however, I met two or three hours weekly with Mrs. Williams for a period of three months at the administrative offices of the V N A. We were joined every two weeks by the mental health consultant.

Before leaving I wanted also to make structurally clear the decision-making process between the Center and the V N A. Internally, the Center had evolved what I would call a dynamic rather than hierarchical arrangement for decision-making. Visually, this arrangement would look like interlacing rings rather than a pyramid: each group of participants (whether those in the four children's clubs, the prenatal or birth-control clinic patients, parents or mothers groups, ad hoc or permanent neighborhood groups) would decide among themselves their own activities. When they wanted program changes they would convey their suggestions through their group sponsor (as Ann or Bernard or Mrs. Jefferson for the clubs, or through Johnnie for the clinic groups, or through Linda for the day care parents, or through Mary Louise for the neighborhood groups) to the Center staff group. There the final decisions would be made. On the whole, the pattern personalized the operation of the Center, since the staff tended to identify with the neighborhood.

But during the transition period as my time to leave drew near, I sensed the staff was dubious about the ultimate link between their "final" decisions and the administration of the V N A, which held the purse strings and managed contractual arrangements with health service agencies. What would happen if their new supervisor did not agree with them? After six months they did not feel confident about what they knew of her, partly because of their own prejudices about "educated" Negroes who had "made it," partly because she was ambivalent about whether her primary identity was "black" and therefore akin to the Center, or "professional" and thus allied to the V N A.

So I made the question explicit with Linda. I asked specifically: would they want the prerogative, officially, to go to the executive director of the V N A if that seemed necessary to them? After two weeks of discussion among themselves, they made their decision: they would work out any disagreements they had with Mrs. Williams among themselves. Somehow my suggestion had implied that they needed to go to whitey in order to settle their problems, even problems with the supervisor who would communicate them to whitey. Having seen it that way, their decision reflected their determination to be self-reliant, it proclaimed a desire for independence. I was pleased with that. At the same time, it precluded a clear channel for appeal—which could frustrate them in the future. Nevertheless, they had decided. I held my breath for them.

Although preparations for transition were complex, they were much simpler than those going on inside of us. In midwinter, I spoke with some of the staff individually about my leaving, both to allow them to react, and to give them time to think about possible changes in the internal organization of the Center. I wanted them to be free to express their doubts and fears, and to look at the whys. But I was torn inside. I wanted them to miss me, to feel a sense of loss. But I wanted also for them to feel a sense of growth in themselves, that I could now go, that they no longer needed me. During the many hours of talking with them individually, listening to the ambivalences, I did not let myself express to them the sense of loss that I was feeling.

I wanted them to focus on melding new relationships, and to express their feelings to each other. I could feel them trying, each in his own way. At one point I, in effect, refused to talk with Mary Louise privately until she began to say what she felt about the transition and about Carlene Williams in front of Carlene and me. What I did was arrange for the three of us to meet together regularly. But I could recognize the puzzlement and pain behind those seemingly vacuous eyes. After a couple of weeks I followed her downstairs to the food cellar and explained not only what I was doing and why—she knew too that she had to try to talk openly with Carlene— but also how hard, how painful, it was for me to do it.

Individually, they let me know when it was time to "announce" my leaving to the staff as a whole, even though, of course, each of them already knew. But it was important to say it to them together. I had spent hours telling them in my head. I wanted to tell them what beautiful people they were, and what beautiful complexities, what unending dimensions to reality had come to my awareness because of them. But I did not, directly.

At the staff meeting, after their initial responses to my "announcement," Linda, rightly enough, shifted the emphasis to them with a statement on the meaning of black power. She could understand that the Center and they could no longer have a white "head"; that the Center could not, even on a symbolic level, perpetuate the pattern so common among the organizations of our society of the white leader and black followers. Linda's statement concentrated their energies, and I did not want to fragment those energies again by focusing on myself, nor take the chance of breaking into tears.

They asked me what I was going to do after I left, what I wanted to do most. I said I wanted to write about them. I wanted to let people in my "category" know what they were like. To my surprise and pleasure, they asked me to use their names, even if I was going to tell the "bad" things. "After all," said Johnnie, "we make mistakes like everyone else; then people will know that we're human too." And they blessed my departure with, in Linda's words, "If y'all want to write, that's what you ought to do. Everyone ought to do what will make them happiest."

Epilogue

Health is wholeness, unfolding.

It is pink skin covering a wound.
It is a book in the hand of the ghetto-dweller,
    and soul music on the lips of the suburbanite.
It is the preschooler's first whoop in day care.
It is knowing,
    not only *I* and *You*
    but *We*.

Health is wholeness, unfolding.

And it is present
Only when we continue to seek
    in ourselves, in our institutions,
    together with others,
A sharing which is significant,
    in the possibilities of man,
A growing awareness of self,
And the feeling of self-worth
    which is the result.

Notes

I. SEARCH FOR COHERENCE

1. Nancy Milio, " 'Ideal' Maternity Behavior as a Pattern Which Reflects the Middle-Class (Dominant Culture) Orientation." (Unpublished master's thesis, Dept. of Sociology, Wayne State University, Detroit, 1965), Appendix A, Table 29.

2. Family income was 20 percent less than for the "average" Detroit family; number of persons per household was 26 percent more than the average; average years of education was less than nine; deaths from child-bearing, prematurity, infections, and other acute and chronic diseases were rising at an accelerating rate; the proportion of usable income (after food, clothing, and shelter) was less than one-fourth of what was left for the average Detroit family. N. Milio, *The Changing Character of a Community: The Threshold of Poverty* (Detroit Visiting Nurse Association, 1964), pp. 6–11. These figures are continuing in the same direction; i.e., the gap is widening between these families and the "average" family.

3. They had 50 percent more children per family, and their infants died at a 17 percent faster rate than did those of the average Detroit family, and almost 60 percent faster than those of the average white family. The proportion of people over sixty-five was increasing, and their death rates from heart disease and cancer were increasing more rapidly than for Detroit as a whole. *Ibid.*, pp. 10, 11, and Statistical Summary, pp. 3 and 5.

4. The Constitution, Eastern Community Council, Detroit, June, 1960.

5. "Program Summary: The Detroit Great Cities School Improvement Project," November 2, 1962.

6. Written communication from the director of the Research Institute, Presbytery of Detroit, April 2, 1962.

7. The Constitution, East Side Improvement Association, Detroit, June, 1963.

8. Detroit Housing Commission, "Neighborhood Conservation Projects," 1962.

9. Economic Opportunity Act of 1964, Title II A, Section 202a, U. S. Congress.

10. Anthony Riply, "Detroit's Militant Rights Groups Aim for Political Power," *The Detroit News*, February 28, 1965.

11. "Community Proposal for the TAP Program," Adult Community

Movement for Equality and Affiliated Block Organizations, Detroit, February, 1965.

12. "A Decentralized, Multiple-Approach Project for Meeting the Maternal and Child Health Aspects of Problems in a Deprived Neighborhood," Detroit Visiting Nurse Association, April 27, 1964.

13. William Strickland, "American and Civil Rights," *Freedom North,* a publication of the Northern Student Movement, 2 (January, 1966), pp. 3–9.

14. "Friends of N S M Statement of Purpose," Detroit, January, 1966.

15. Frances Reissman Cousens, "Indigenous Leadership: A Study of Perception and Participation in Two Lower-Class Neighborhood Organizations" (unpublished doctoral dissertation, Wayne State University, Detroit, 1962).

II. FORMATION OF A MATRIX

1. Two cultural strands among Black people, those who accept white middle-class ways (the "acculturated") and those who conform superficially to the white world (the "externally adapted"), exist *at all income levels.* See Jessie Bernard, *Marriage and Family among Negroes* (Englewood Cliffs, N. J.: Prentice-Hall, Inc., 1966), pp. 27–67.

2. A thorough discussion of the philosophical, historical, and cultural bases for these questions are found in F. S. C. Northrop's *The Meeting of East and West* (New York: The Macmillan Co., 1946; Macmillan Paperbacks Edition, 1960), and, in the area of political-economics (the "red/expert" dilemma), in Franz Schurmann, *Ideology and Organization in Communist China* (Berkeley, Calif.: University of California Press, 1966), Sec. I.

3. See Philip Selznick "Critical Decisions in Organizational Development," in *Complex Organizations,* Amitai Etzioni, Ed. (New York: Holt, Rinehart, and Winston, 1961), pp. 355–63.

III. DISCOVERING THE POSSIBLE

1. This requirement was not rigidly enforced for mothers who had many children or many problems at home. The only eligibility requirement was residence within an approximately mile-square area of the Center.

2. Of the preschoolers (three and a half to five years) enrolled during the first year, a total of fifty-two (fifteen at a time),
65 percent had no regular physician or clinic
54 percent had never been immunized
64 percent came from families having three or more children.

Thirty-four of their mothers participated in the program.

3. Paid $15 per hour, one or two hours a week. He had just begun his private practice.

4. Usually, pregnant women from the neighborhood would get their initial prenatal examination (including laboratory procedures) through the obstetrical service of a downtown hospital; it was receiving federal funds for the maternity care of low-income women. The hospital would then allow the women who did not have apparent medical or obstetrical complications to go to Mom and Tots for their monthly examinations until delivery. The patients were delivered at the hospital and later received their six-week postnatal examination there.

5. Birth defects, including mental retardation, are reduced four-fold when pregnancies are more than fifteen months apart. Paul Todd, chief executive officer, Planned Parenthood-World Population, Testimony to Senate Finance Committee on Social Security Amendments, H.R. 12080 (Washington, D.C., September 22, 1967).

6. Some of the answers of the first seventy-six patients, in comparison with eighty-five public health nurses were:

	Patients (Percent)	Nurses (Percent)
Beginning prenatal care:		
As soon as pregnancy is known	71	96
Between 3 and 6 mos.	25	4
Just before delivery	4	0
Prenatal care begun when last pregnant		(out of 40)
1–3 mos.	46	93
4–6 mos.	33	7
7–9 mos.	11	0
No answer	11	0
Should you plan each child?		
Yes	89	94
Did you plan your last baby?		(out of 40)
Yes	13	50
Best family planning methods:		
Pill or IUD	29	40
Other artificial methods	45	41
Abstinence	3	14
"Be careful"	7	0
Did not know	17	5

	Patients *(Percent)*	Nurses *(Percent)*
Sources for birth-control supplies:		
Physician or clinic	64	88
Drugstore	5	5
Did not know	33	7
When do you usually go to the doctor?		
	(out of 35)	
Regularly	29	78
When sick	66	25
Do not go	0	4
If you had $15 left out of your paycheck and		
a) the light bill was due	3	5
b) your child needed medicine	91	93
c) you were pregnant but had not gone to the doctor yet	3	0
d) there was a sale on for TV's	0	0
What would you do?		
If you were fixing dinner one evening and		
a) a friend called and said you had a good chance of getting a job if you applied before the store closes	6	6
b) your husband came home hungry	37	20
c) your child came home sick	54	68
What would you take care of first?		
If you had a free afternoon and could		
a) rest	14	14
b) take your child to the park	3	9
c) get a check-up	3	5
d) take your child for his shots	77	58
What would you do?		

These answers reveal a basic area of agreement between middle-income nurses and low-income patients on the importance of the well-being of children. Although many studies have demonstrated wide differences in the areas of their general interests and use of leisure time, this appears not to be so where small children are concerned. When brought to the attention of low-income mothers, the health of children is as important to them as it is to the nurses whose job it is to promote health.

The point of divergence appears to come regarding *when* health care is sought. This difference may result from (1) variant perceptions of sickness and the purposes of health care (i.e., whether ideally preventive or curative in nature), (2) the relative possibility of seeking health care in the light of priorities defined by one's life situation, and (3) the relative difference in institutionalized deterrents in the system of health-care services presented to various socio-economic groups. . . .

Merely "teaching the patient what she should do" has little meaning and has little effect on patient behavior, as recent studies have found. . . .

Providing health services to low-income patients in a manner that is acceptable within their socio-cultural setting should result in an increased use of services. This then might eventually lead to changes in their perception of how it feels to be "sick" or "healthy." However, utilization of services will continue to be limited insofar as other concrete, emergent needs, inherent in the low-income context, take priority for the time, energy, and money of low-income people. N. Milio, "Value Emphases Regarding Certain Health Care Practices among Indigent Prenatal Patients and Public Health Nurses" (Detroit Visiting Nurse Association, June, 1967).

7. The rationale for this is that the chances for death among nonwhite babies compared to white babies is 50 percent greater at birth, 200 percent greater by the end of the first week of life, and 300 percent greater between the third and eighth months of life (National Center for Health Statistics, *Vital and Health Statistics: Infant and Prenatal Mortality in the U. S.*, Series 3, No. 4, U.S. Dept. of Health, Education, and Welfare, Washington, D.C., October, 1965, p. 15). Visits to the home were made following delivery, when the mother would have greatest difficulty leaving the house. Prenatal home visits were not made, except on requests. But no requests were ever made.

8. Of the first fifty-one prenatal patients (April 1966–January, 1967)—the period prior to the funding crisis—their ages were:

	Percent
Under 17	8
17–24	55
25–34	33
35 and over	4
	100

their number of previous pregnancies were:

	Percent
1	24
2–4	47
5 or more	29
	100

their marital status was:

	Percent
single	26
married	55
separated or divorced	20
	100

Six months following delivery for these fifty-one women:

84 percent were using a child-spacing method (the pill or intrauterine device—IUD).

43 percent of their babies had been immunized and another 20 percent had appointments for a medical evaluation and immunizations.

N. Milio, "The Child-Bearing Phase of Maternity: A Comparison of Traditional and Neighborhood Oriented Patterns of Prenatal Care" (Detroit Visiting Nurse Association, November, 1967).

9. During the first six months of the family-planning clinic (November, 1966–March, 1967) the average rate of new patients coming per month was twenty. About one-third came from families whose income was $75 or more per week.

During the six-month period of November, 1967–March, 1968, the average rate of new patients coming per month was forty. Again, about one-third had a family income of $75 or more per week. The total active case load reached five hundred in March, 1968.

10. Later, in July, 1967, when OEO family-planning funds became available, all services were free of charge to women living in the area.

11. This policy was changed in July, 1967.

12. Adapted from *Testing the Aide's Skills with Children* (New York: National League for Nursing, 1967).

13. Each Club had one of its sessions a month centered on "health" (broadly defined). This was led by a community health nurse, a practical nurse, or other "official" health worker.

14. Used by permission from the author.

15. The history and use of indirection from the days of African slavery and slavery in America is discussed by Melville Herskovits in *The Myth of the Negro Past* (Boston: Beacon Press, 1958), pp. 154–58.
16. From a taped talk at the annual meeting of the Detroit VNA, February, 1967.

IV. BARRIERS

1. Most charges were dropped before they were released on bond. The disposition of the "inciting to riot" charges was "decision pending trial at a later date" ("Status of A A Y M-N S M Arrests," mimeo, People against Racism, Detroit, September 22, 1966). The disturbance was not legally considered a riot; no convictions were made by March 4, 1967 (*The Detroit News*, March 4, 1967). On May 29, 1968, a newscast reported that two of the men were convicted of "obstructing police."
2. The Mom and Tots Center had a provisional license for day care because Mertus Butler had only one rather than two years of college course work.
3. These projects were funded under the Social Security Amendments of 1963 (Maternity and Infant Care) and 1965 (Children and Youth).

VI. CONVULSION

1. N. Milio, "The Detroit Riot," *American Journal of Nursing*, 68 (March, 1968), p. 509.
2. This designation often, but not always, saved stores from being looted or burned.
3. The Center also agreed to be an emergency day-care facility as requested by United Community Services.
4. "The Black Star Cooperative," Black Star Co-op, Inc., Detroit, 1967.
5. The foregoing is based on an article by N. Milio, "Untouched in the Holocaust," *American Journal of Nursing*, 68 (March, 1968), pp. 508–9.
6. Philip Meyer, "The Rioter—and What Sets Him Apart," *Detroit Free Press*, August 20, 1967.
   Further analysis of the Detroit riot appeared in a supplement to *Trans-action*, September–October, 1967 (St. Louis, Mo., Washington University).
7. Russell Dynes and E. L. Quarantelli, "What Looting in Civil Disturbances Really Means," *Trans-action*, May, 1968, pp. 13–14.

VII. STRENGTHENING THE MATRIX

1. Funds for these changes were from the supporters of the Center who came to the fore during the months of its financial and organizational crises (November, 1966 to July, 1967; see Part V). The Mom and Tots Center entered the formalization phase of its development about eighteen months after its inception. During the year following the resumption of funding under OEO (from July 1, 1967), certain procedures were routinized, assuring its continuity as an ongoing organization under the umbrella of the VNA, to end, in effect, its hand-to-mouth, day-to-day, existence.

   Financially, 80 percent of budgeted funds were assured from OEO through August, 1969, and were renewable on an annual basis. The remaining 20 percent of the budget, as required under OEO, was reasonably assured from local sources: clubs, churches, community groups, as well as Planned Parenthood and Kirwood General Hospital (one hospital participating in the prenatal care program). These latter two were, by 1968, submitting to the VNA their components of the Mom and Tots budget. The VNA Board of Trustees through its Special Projects Committee began in the spring of 1968 a quarterly newsletter, *The Sounds of Mom and Tots*, which was mailed to contributors.

   In terms of its organizational relationship to the VNA, the Center had all supplies which were ordered outside the neighborhood billed to the main office of the VNA. Neighborhood purchases were made in cash. The reimbursement procedure as well as the payroll was maintained by the Center's secretary directly with the main office. She also reported monthly statistics to the clerical staff of the main office.

   In the fall of 1967 the Center was represented at the bi-monthly VNA administrative-supervisory meetings. Personnel policies for the Mom and Tots staff were also brought into line with those of the rest of the VNA.

   A final step in the organizational development of the Center was dissolving its "project" status by routinizing the procedures indicated here and by replacing the project director with a supervisor.

2. Grace and James Boggs, "Detroit: Birth of A Nation," *The National Guardian*, October 7, 1967.

3. Negro mothers are said to cultivate and reinforce a submerged and ill-defined identity in male children, one which society has forced on Negro men for generations, a "negative" recognition. See Erik Erikson, *Identity: Youth and Crisis* (New York: W. W. Norton and Co., 1968), Chapter 8.

4. Inge and Sten Hegeler, *An ABZ of Love* (Copenhagen, Denmark: Chr. Erichsen's Forlag, 1963). Now available in paperback.
5. M.P.H.—master of public health.
6. Basic sources used for the discussion of human sexuality at the Center were Ruth and Edward Brecher, Eds., *An Analysis of Human Sexual Response* (New York: New American Library, Signet Paperback, 1966); Erich Fromm, *The Art of Loving* (New York: Harper and Row, 1956); Inge and Sten Hegeler, *An ABZ of Love*, (Copenhagen, Denmark: Chr. Erichsen's Forlag, 1963); Ira Reiss, Ed., "The Sexual Renaissance in America," *Journal of Social Issues*, 22 (April, 1966).
7. There is a wisely cautious discussion of the meaning of "soul" by Ulf Hannerz in *Trans-action*, July–August, 1968, with several articles criticizing what we think we know about black people in the United States, "Negroes in the New World."

VIII. WHOLENESS UNFOLDING

1. This chapter illustrates, among other things, the aspect of organizational development in which the core staff, having matured in their roles, perform the essential task of orienting newcomers (see Philip Selznick, "Critical Decisions in Organizational Development," in *Complex Organizations*, Amitai Etzioni, Ed. (New York: Holt, Rinehart, and Winston, 1961).
2. All job descriptions were written two years after the Center began, after agreement was reached among the staff on each person's responsibilities. Although certain functions were thus circumscribed, their responsibilities continued, of course, to overlap and evolve, helping to preserve an essential dynamic in the Center. New organizations need to be cautious about premature formalization of positions and procedures, since this has been found to limit openendedness and seal off leadership (see *ibid.*). These are the positions as they evolved:

Driver (Mr. Hatt)

1. Transport patients under the direction of Community Worker.
2. Report hourly by phone to the Center when away from the Center.
3. Maintain VW station wagon—inspections, car wash, gas.
4. Turn in mileage, maintenance receipts, and gas bill monthly to secretary.
5. Perform general maintenance at Mom and Tots as time allows under direction of Community Worker.

Clinic Assistant (Johnnie West)

1. Help plan prenatal clinic discussions with community health nurse and practical nurse.
2. Lead group discussions in prenatal and family planning clinics.
3. Help prepare prenatal patients for examinations before physician arrives.
4. Help prepare prenatal charts and rooms for clinic.
5. Help maintain bulletin boards and kitchens.
6. Instruct home visitors about information for door-to-door contacts.
7. See that appointments obtained by home visitors are correctly reported.
8. Report working time of home visitors to the secretary.
9. Help develop audio-visual materials.

Secretary (Ada Dixon)

1. Do general typing.
2. Answer telephone.
3. Share in making appointments.
4. Maintain time cards.
5. Maintain petty cash disbursement and receipts.
6. Receive day-care fees from day-care supervisor.
7. Record monthly statistical summary and recording on follow-up cards.
8. Order office supplies from V N A main office.
9. Compile data for evaluation as necessary.

Day-Care Supervisor (Linda MacKay)

1. Lead in planning daily activities.
2. Lead daily review of day-care program.
3. Supervise day-care staff.
4. Help supervise meal planning, buying, and preparation.
5. Lead and plan with staff for "inservice education," including attendance at workshops.
6. Plan excursions for children.
7. Interview and orient new mothers to day care.
8. Schedule mothers in staffing day care.
9. Set and collect fees with working mothers.
10. Order supplies and equipment.
11. Maintain day-care cash budget.
12. Work with community health nurse to include teaching for preschoolers and staff.
13. Share in planning and leading Parents Club meetings.
14. Share in programs affecting entire Center.
15. Encourage as much as possible the involvement of staff and

neighborhood women in planning and carrying out work and children's activities.

Community Worker (Mary Louise Moore)

1. Maintain close contact with community groups, including ESVID, CESSA, block clubs, churches, schools, etc.
2. See that the Center programs become known to neighborhood via handbills and other means.
3. Plan and coordinate general activities directed to the neighborhood as a whole, e.g., seasonal programs, variety night, and films.
4. Maintain sponsors for children's groups.
5. Conduct transportation program.
6. Supervise driver and housekeeper.
7. See that building stays in good repair.
8. Make necessary contacts with landlord.

3. Planned Parenthood issued a new Policy Statement in June, 1967. It was in effect immediately at the Center:
We believe in responsible parenthood as necessary for stable family life, which is the nucleus of any community. We believe that every child born should be welcome and that every woman has the right and responsibility to plan for her babies. We are deeply concerned that she have some alternative beyond seeking illegal abortion or giving birth to an unwanted child. For these reasons our policy is to receive in our clinic all women who request and need our services, as follows:
1. Any woman of any age who is married.
2. Any woman under the age of twenty-one who has had a pregnancy and who signs a certification of age provided by Planned Parenthood.
3. Any woman over age of twenty-one who signs the certification of age form.
4. Any woman within six months of marriage who signs a statement of intent to marry. Confirmation of the wedding date must be submitted within the six months. If confirmation is not received, service will be given in accordance with Items 2, 3, and/or 5.
5. An unmarried girl under twenty-one who has never been pregnant and is not getting married must have a parent or guardian's written permission witnessed by a member of the Planned Parenthood League staff. When parents are deceased or cannot be located and there is no legal guardian, this girl may be accepted as a patient on referral by a qualified representative of a recognized public or private agency or other professional persons.